For Reuben and Uma – to your futures.

CONTENTS

Preface 6

Why I wrote this book 8

Before we begin: How to use this book .... .14

I. THE FOUNDATIONS .... .17

Behaviours and Biology .... .18

Systems and symptoms .... .36

II. THE ASPIRATIONS .... .55

'I want more energy' .... .57

'I want better digestion' .... .74

'I want to beat those aches and pains' .... .83

'I want to improve my mood, and feel calm and focused' ..... .93

'I want to deal with these mystery symptoms' .... .110

'I want a sharper memory' .... .120

'I want to stop being ill all the time' .... .138

'I just want to feel like I used to' .... .145

III. THE FIXES 155

Putting it all together 156

Diet 168

Exercise: Movement and posture 176

Sleep 190

Stress. 195

Daily prevention hacks. 200

Conclusion: A few final words and the beauty of science . . . 205

IV. YOUR HEALTH FIX 211

Glossary. 228

Endnotes. 240

Index 246

Acknowledgements. 254

Preface

I am writing this book during another extraordinary year in our lives. Personally and professionally, I cannot think of a tougher time to have lived through.

The world has changed in the space of three years. Like so many of us, I have had to make some big changes to my life in order to survive, let alone thrive. Working at a sometimes unsustainable pace, prioritising my time to make room for what is really important, getting rid of negative forces from my life, and thinking carefully about my purpose were all in the mix.

Many musings from this book can be found on my podcast, *Saving Lives in Slow Motion*, the feedback for which I have been greatly humbled by. If you happen to have listened to it, then you will have already heard some of my ramblings about various parts of this book. The podcast vignettes hopefully made sense, but of course there were pieces that were intentionally missing. Well, *voilà* – your jigsaw is now complete.

To protect the privacy and confidentiality of actual patients, I have combined features of several cases in each chapter and disguised any identifying information in each case. Those patients and their family stories that feature in this book should be regarded as fictional.

I have done my best to bring you what you need to either get started on or continue with your **Health Fix** journey. Some people will need a total reset, some a push, others will possibly resume after a pause.

Despite the strap line, there is no magic eight-week plan with any kind of curated timetable, no fads, no judgement and no unnecessary gloss. You will soon realise that the method laid out in this book is tailored to you. In my experience, people tend to feel better within eight weeks, often sooner.

I hope the book's foundations will strengthen you, that the stories will inspire you and that *The Health Fix* will transform your life for the better.

Dr Ayan Panja
St Albans, Hertfordshire, UK
June 2022

"True healing is not the fixing of the broken, but the rediscovery of the unbroken."
Jeff Foster

Why I wrote this book

About eight years ago, my health was at an all-time low. I was unable to think straight, my memory was failing and I kept falling asleep during the day. I couldn't digest my food properly, my joints ached on most days and I was generally irritable and unhappy. On some days, I could hardly function. I remember walking into the coffee shop next door to my surgery one morning and not being able to place an order as my brain seemed incapable of making a simple decision.

Like most people who find themselves just not feeling well (as opposed to suddenly falling ill), it had all crept up on me in slow motion. It took me the best part of six months to figure out why I was so broken – and once I finally worked it out, I felt human again after eight weeks.

The answers lay not in medical interventions, but changes to my lifestyle. Despite seeing patients, day in, day out, I had somehow managed to take my eye off the ball with my own health, getting caught up in the throes of my busy work and family life, coupled with hitting the age of forty.

'Honestly, mate, it all falls apart at forty,' my friends were telling me at the time – but it really was more than that.

The final straw was when I met one of my best friends for dinner in London, and he said, 'You OK, mate? You look fucked...'

What the heck had happened to me? And how could I fix myself?

My own symptoms sent me on a journey that has changed my life and the lives of many others. So far I have had thirty years' worth of learning, clinical practice and teaching since I started medical school, and they have helped me build the framework and the tools I used to claim my health back. I am sharing this framework and these tools in this book. As you have probably guessed by the title, I managed to fix my health to a point where I could carry on enjoying my life to the full, and I hope that soon you will be able to do the same for yourself and your loved ones.

THE MISSION

I sometimes can't believe I am having to write a book like this. The concept of 'health is wealth' is one that only dawns on us either when things go wrong or as we get older. When you were fourteen years old, you may have thought of someone who was forty or fifty as 'quite old'. I am almost fifty myself now, but in my head I feel that my parents and their friends are still fifty (Mum is now nearer eighty, as it goes).

There is no arguing with the fact that as we age, we become more likely to develop long-term conditions.[1]

The truth is, time flies, and our biological functions slowly decline with time as our cells undergo more damage. As one of our ex-students once said to me as though it were some kind of revelation, 'More stuff happens to people as they get older, doesn't it?' When it comes to maximising health, I like to think of myself as Bill Gates's 'lazy employee'.

"I choose a lazy person to do a hard job. Because a lazy person will find an easy way to do it."
Bill Gates[2]

I want to stay as well as I can and enjoy my life for as long as I can, with minimum fuss. And this is what I want to share with you.

THE PROBLEM

The landscape of our health is constantly changing. By that, I mean our world at large: air pollution, soil quality, farming practices, climate change, our exposure to plastics, chemicals or radiation, the influence of social media, our reliance on technology, pandemic viruses... the list of things that can disrupt our health continues to evolve.[3]

The trouble is that because this all happens so innocuously, the chances are you won't notice the invisible effects that these factors – and your own habits – are having on your health; that is, until you start to get symptoms or your health declines.

To put it another way, you don't just wake up one day with a condition like irritable bowel syndrome, chronic lung disease, arthritis, multiple sclerosis, depression, Alzheimer's disease or type 2 diabetes. It takes months, sometimes years, of increasing dysfunction in the body's biological systems for these conditions to manifest. We will explore this further later on in the book.

The other problem we are presented with right now is the challenges facing the medical profession. As doctors, we genuinely do our best to help patients, based on the most up-to-date scientific evidence from population studies and trials, as we grapple with increasing levels of illness.[4] Yet the resources and tools we have to hand are often not the right ones to deal with the symptoms that are presented to us. This is particularly the case when it comes to treating individuals who come to us seeking help with vague, medically unexplained or non-emergency symptoms, including headaches, bloating, pain or fatigue.[5] There is a disconnect, a palpable gap, with which both doctors and patients are familiar, and what is needed is a fresh, sustainable and non-faddish approach.

There are so many books out there about habits, health, self-help and improvement. The medical and scientific community are often sceptical about these publications, which often promise a better life. Many of them seem to contain quite a lot of overlapping content. Some are by celebrities or influencers with lived experience; others are written by those in the scientific community themselves.

With some of these publications, there is often an element of reinventing the wheel but with different spokes. I am all for scepticism as it helps us to call out hokum and snake oil, but we must also acknowledge that there is so much we still don't understand in both science and medicine.

The other thing you may have noticed is that those who are eminent in their fields of science or humanities often put out content that chimes with that found in the lay-authored books, because their disciplines or areas of scientific or social research prove that these practices 'work'. It could be anything from high intensity training, ice baths, forest bathing or using certain behavioural techniques. I have a lot of time for a number of academic experts writing in the field of health, including (at the time of writing), Tim Spector (epidemiology),[6] and Satchidananda Panda (regulatory biology).[7] Whatever their field, there is a lot of synergy in their output, whether it be about the brain, the gut, our habits or their own original research. As this book unfolds, you will see why.

My view is that, as patients, we have the power to make changes, but need some direction when things are not going the right way. With *The Health Fix*, my offering is neither that of a researcher or an academic professor, but nor is it simply my own lay views. I have the lived experience of being a patient, but I have also treated thousands of people over the years as a doctor. In order to practise medicine, one must keep up with the latest science. My expertise involves taking the patient's story and using the available science and evidence to formulate an individual plan with them that is tailored to them alone.

Where people have access to it, modern medicine is rather impressive, particularly when it comes to procedures or protocols, such as surgically cutting out disease, or prescribing medication for long-term conditions. Medics are near enough amazing at dealing with acute presentations, such as trauma, life-threatening infections, heart attacks and strokes. But we do tend to struggle with the more nebulous, undefined, interpretive work[8] involving complaints such as recurrent illness,* the rise in mental health distress, or conditions that seem to lack particularly effective treatments. Of the latter, the one that has been on my mind the most in the last year has been 'long COVID'. We have struggled as a profession to help those afflicted with this syndrome, which often manifests as a cluster of debilitating symptoms. In my experience, the best campaigners for unmet needs are often doctors who are also patients.

. . .

---

* I am mindful that, in some parts of the world, there are obvious factors like poor sanitation that claim lives from diarrhoeal disease and respiratory illnesses on a daily basis.[9]

The paradox of modern medicine hit me when I realised that my work as a hospital doctor had enabled me to save lives in emergencies, but when I was faced with a chap who came in and said, 'Doctor, I get this horrible constant shaking feeling every day, but it's just on the inside, if you get what I mean – what do you think it could be?', I realised I really hadn't a clue about the reasons behind a lot of people's symptoms and it was often easy to cast them into that well of uncertainty called 'medically unexplained symptoms'.[10]

When they hear the story of my own illness, as I described it earlier, many of my doctor friends try to pin it all down to one diagnosis, because that's how we are trained:

'Maybe you were depressed?'

'Maybe you had IBS for a bit, and it just got better?'

'Maybe you've got Lyme disease?'

They were trying to give me a diagnosis or a label. In reality, multiple symptoms indicate some kind of system malfunction – that system being our own human biology.[11]

In order to change and control our biology, we need to look at the inputs that affect it and manipulate them to our advantage.

Before we begin: How to use this book

I am not a psychologist, but as a general practitioner, I would say this book is really as much about you understanding yourself as it is about any kind of framework I'll be sharing with you. It will give you a toolkit that you will be able to use time and time again.

The book is composed of three main sections:

The Foundations

The Aspirations

The Fixes

The Foundations section is all about our *behaviours* and our *biology*. This is an essential tour of the key aspects of our mental and physical processes; in essence, it's about 'what makes us tick' as human beings.

The Aspirations section is a collection of real-world *Health Fix* cases, covering patients' stories on emotional, physical and scientific levels. The cases represent the most common 'health wishes' I have come across over my twenty-four years of clinical work as a qualified doctor.

The Fixes are the strategies, tools and, dare I say it, hacks that you can use to improve your health. This section will also show you how you can put it all together for yourself.

Already, some readers might be tempted to jump ahead to this last section, but the book won't work for you if you do that. The idea of **The Health Fix** is that it really works around you as an individual, and the Fixes you'll adopt will vary depending on your own symptoms and needs.

There are a number of concepts that I hope will stay with you. Shortly, you will explore the **IDEAL** framework, which allows you to change behaviours.

Soon after that, you will come across the **Health Loop**. This is at the core of how you will 'fix' many of your issues, and lays out your current health in a way that you may not have thought about before, focusing on eight key factors.

You will then write your own **Lifestyle Prescription**, which will most likely lead you to a phenomenon called the **Drawstring Effect**, where everything literally tightens up and comes together.

There are also sections throughout called **Deep Dives**, where I expand on the science behind the stories I've shared. In addition, you will learn about the subtle power of **How, What and When**, as well as when to **Drill Down and Diary Up**.

Just let this wash over you for now, much like the overture at the start of a musical or an opera when the orchestra plays a few bars from each song, so that everything seems oddly familiar when you come across them later.

Now, let us begin.

I

THE
FOUNDATIONS

"The noblest pleasure is the joy of understanding."
Leonardo da Vinci

8

BEHAVIOURS
AND BIOLOGY

Twenty-four hours a day, the body's biological processes continue to keep us alive. During our waking hours, our behavioural processes join in and our days become a stream of continuous biological and behavioural actions. These actions have consequences that usually occur without much conscious thought. In simple terms, it is the mind and body working together.

Let's start by taking a look at behaviour, and in particular how it relates to our health. Our brains are constantly receiving information and processing it, so it is important to think about what makes us tick if we are going to then use it to our advantage.

When it comes to health, simply using willpower or being told what to do by your family, friends, therapist, nurse, doctor or influencer will not work for a lot of people. Just think about how hard it can be to stop smoking or to cut down your sugar intake, or to start a new healthy habit, like taking up regular exercise for the first time. In order to make useful changes in your life, the bottom line is that you need to be able to change your behaviours.

Understanding our behaviours and how to change them

Most of our behaviours are learned from watching or reacting to the world around us. Slowly but surely, over time, these behaviours become ingrained in us, in the same way that most children do what their parents *do*, not necessarily what they *say*. In fact, our childhood experiences and how we were parented have a surprising amount of influence on our behaviour as adults.[12]

What fascinates me is that not only are our behaviours important to our health and wellbeing, they also absolutely define us. How many times do you find yourself saying something like, 'My boyfriend's just not the kind of person to ever take up running... he's so lazy.' Where does that kind of statement or judgement come from? It's based on the boyfriend's historical behaviours, habits and track record (or lack of – forgive the pun), all of which suggest to you, and possibly the rest of the world, that he's not the kind of person who will take up running.

This can be quite damaging, not least because it can lead us to totally write someone off. And if that someone starts to believe what other people say, that in itself can be a barrier to change, becoming what psychologists call a 'false belief'.[13]

I remember saying at a big family dinner some years ago that I might run the Great Wall Marathon in China, as a local friend had mooted it. Everyone fell about laughing as if I had told them a Spike Milligan joke.

'Sorry. What's so funny?' I barked.

'You can't even run five kilometres! What was it last time? You were going to join that tennis club? Or was it that you were *definitely* taking up golf this year? Hmm, yeah – how did that all turn out again?'

The point is, they had made a judgement based on my past behaviours, or my track record, if you like. I am a dreamer, for sure.

When I was a teenager, my father used to tell me: 'I know you better than you know yourself.'

What dad really meant by that rather forthright statement was that he knew my behaviours all too well.

Despite being defined by our behaviours and habits, the good news is that we can change these. A leopard *can* change its spots. We just need to work out how to change. But first, we really need buy-in as to *why* it is necessary to change in the first place.

Most of us have some repetitive behaviours, which are effectively habits, and habits become automatic. For instance, you might pick up your phone first thing each morning and read the same daily news feeds, or you might take a shower at the same time each day, or go to the same shops each week, or take the same route to work every morning.

What's all this got to do with your health?

Well, there are some behaviours or habits that are harmful and easy to recognise as problematic, especially if they become 'automatic' (such as smoking) – but there are other harmful habits that might not be so obvious.

This means two things need to happen:

1. Identifying and understanding if and why a habit is causing you harm.

2. Changing that habit.

A quick word on behavioural theory

According to Stanford's Professor B. J. Fogg, a world-leading behaviour-change expert, there are three elements that need to come together to enable you to change a behaviour or habit: motivation, ability and a prompt. Fogg calls 'B=MAP':[14]

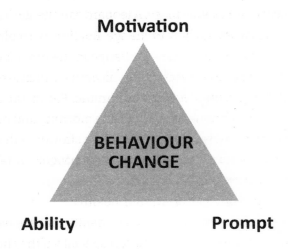

(Credit: B. J. Fogg)

What does this actually mean?

Well, in order to create behaviour change:

• We need to be sufficiently **motivated** to make a change.

• We need to have the **ability** to do it.

• We need a **prompt** to turn it into an action.

Let's take a common example. You've been thinking about taking up running. You're really **motivated** because you want to get into better shape for your wedding. You have the **ability** to do it (i.e. you have all the kit and the time you need). But you just haven't got round to it – in other words, there is no **prompt**. So what can you use to prompt you into action?

The secret is to **make it easy**. Leave your trainers and joggers at the door; leave apples out in the fruit bowl. Much of this is about controlling your environment, as you will see a little later.

Reminders like sticky notes and alarms can be useful as prompts that make you 'do it now', but to really answer this properly, we ought to look at how you might have changed your behaviours previously.

Behavioural theory is all well and good, but having carefully listened to my patients and their stories over many years, I have realised that there are only a handful of real-world reasons that make us change our behaviours. As you read on, take a moment to reflect and see if any of these scenarios sound familiar.

HAPPY ACCIDENTS

This is when something happens totally unintentionally, but has positive consequences. For example, a while back I forgot to have a coffee one morning, and only realised the next day that I hadn't had any caffeine at all for twenty-four hours. I absolutely *love* coffee, by the way – the smell, the taste, making it, slurping it. Like many medics, I had become a bit reliant on it as a junior doctor. But as I hadn't noticed not having it for a whole day, and because I seemed to feel better without it, I decided to see if I could stay off it. As it goes, it was so easy and I felt so much calmer without it.

UNDER ORDERS

This is when external rules or laws temporarily force our habits and curb our behaviours.

Think about the no-smoking signs on a plane, or the way alcohol is not available to drink in certain states or countries. These examples are particularly powerful, as even the most hardened smoker will tell you that she doesn't seem to crave cigarettes on a plane because it's simply not an option. And if beer and wine are not on a menu, then you have to order a soft drink. This kind of external enforcement makes you realise that our minds are very powerful. You really *can* go without a cigarette for fourteen hours if you have to. Somehow, it's easier to follow rules made by others than to enforce your own. Essentially, these situations make it difficult for you to engage in a behaviour because of imposed restrictions.

THE UNTHINKABLE

Tragedy is a brutal leveller. All too often I have heard heart-breaking stories of unexpected loss or illness. A best friend dies of a heart attack, or a loved one gets diagnosed with terminal cancer. These unthinkable events can act as a prompt, often jolting us into making changes that are rooted deeply in fear or purpose.

COMMUNITY SPIRIT

Doing things with others as part of a group – what some people call 'finding their tribe' – can be a great behaviour-change prompt.

Take Parkrun, Weight Watchers or Slimming World; none of them offer any kind of magic pill or potion or Nobel Prize-winning discovery, but they have effectively harnessed the remarkable power of community and understood how it can change behaviours, and so help people change their lives.

FRIENDLY JEALOUSY

Imagine you meet up with a friend you haven't seen in six months. He looks and feels fantastic compared to when you last saw him. You almost can't believe the transformation. He has clearer skin, seems calm and confident, and has clearly improved various aspects of his work and home life. You go home and think, 'I'd like some of that myself.' Your friend is the prompt, especially if you have been thinking about some changes for a while without getting round to making them.

GRASPING THE NETTLE

By this, I mean forcing yourself to do something through sheer bloody-mindedness.

This is really hard work, and only for people who are able to follow their own imposed rules without rhyme or reason. It relies heavily on willpower, which, as I explained earlier, is not a good strategy for everyone.

The happy accident, under orders and to some extent **the unthinkable** are out of our conscious control. This is why they often work without much conscious effort.

Community spirit, **friendly jealousy** and **grasping the nettle** all require that B. J. Fogg triad of **motivation**, **ability** and **prompt**.

Do any of those examples ring true to you? What all of them illustrate is that changing our habits is entirely possible, and even *easy* given the right circumstances. They also involve a level of control.

THE HEALTH FIX

The IDEAL framework

To make it easy, I have come up with a framework called **IDEAL**. Don't worry about having to actively remember this, as you will come across it throughout the book and it will become totally instinctive after a while.

The **IDEAL** framework is a really easy way to start changing your habits.

IDENTIFY what you would like to do (e.g. taking up running; stopping smoking).

DEFINE one or two small changes you can make (e.g. running to work instead of walking; deciding to leave the house without cigarettes).

ENGAGE by preparing and controlling your environment to make change easy (e.g. set out your running kit the night before; make sure you have no cigarettes in the house).

ACTIVATE yourself by sticking your new habit(s) on to an existing one, or use them to replace a bad one. We'll explore this in more detail below.

LOOK BACK at yourself in the mirror and say, 'Hey, you did it. Well done.'

The last one might sound silly. You don't actually need to look in the mirror, but you should pat yourself on the back each time you perform the new habit. It's important to acknowledge your efforts. Think of it as the opposite of being hard on yourself.

By now, I hope this is all beginning to resonate with you as something that is relevant to your health but also doable. Soon, you will be able to change your habits for the better. This may seem nebulous at the moment, but once you've read the next section, which explores our biology, I hope you will see why this section about behaviours was so important.

A IS FOR 'ACTIVATE'

One key factor, again championed by B. J. Fogg, is to add a new habit or behaviour to an existing one. This is what I call 'activate' in the **IDEAL** framework, and the idea is for the new and old habits to feed and encourage each other. New habits are far more likely to 'stick' this way, rather than falling by the wayside after a few weeks, like all those New Year's resolutions.

For instance, if you decide you want to do two press-ups a day or learn a new fact each morning, why not do it straight after something that you already do every single day, like brushing your teeth? Or, if you want to start a weekly outdoor habit, like going for a run, how about doing it just after you put the bins out? After a while, it will become a familiar association: we are familiar with coffee and cake or milk and cookies but how about brushing your teeth and press-ups?

Now imagine the difference between you and your imaginary twin, who has been doing two daily press-ups and learning a new fact every day for ten years. Your twin would be stronger (and better at Christmas quizzes, most likely). But in all seriousness, the point is that even small regular habits and behaviours can give huge rewards if they are carried out regularly and continued. It's all about the power of marginal gains over time, which works much like compound interest. Some benefits are invisible; others are obvious. But if anything should demonstrate why it's worth 'sticking with it', it's this graph:

How habits improve over time

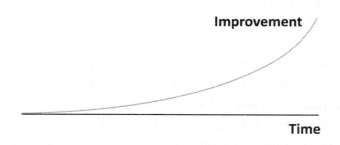

Improvement

Time

Bad habits and managing your monkey brain

How many times have you said to yourself, 'It seemed like a good idea at the time...'? If you stop for a minute and think about any bad habit you might have that you would like to change, have you ever wondered why you still do it even though you know it's bad?

I remember being in a queue for a barbecue buffet in a hotel in Egypt many years ago. I got chatting to a guy called Tom behind me. He was smoking a cigarette and he said, 'This is so stupid. One part of my brain really wants to smoke this fag, but the other part knows it's killing me... what the heck is going on, doc?'

What he was referring to was his 'monkey brain'. We all have this primitive part of our brain (namely the prefrontal cortex and limbic system) which is powerful, impulsive, reactionary and emotional. We need to acknowledge our monkey brain, but also stop it from controlling or hijacking us.

Have you ever felt bad because you snapped at a friend? Or reached for a packet of doughnuts and eaten all of them in one go? Or felt road rage? Don't worry – most of us have. That's our monkey brain at work. All of these things give us a quick hit or fix of something 'without thought'. Often, the actions we take make us feel emotionally or physically terrible, or racked with guilt afterwards.

One of my patients from years ago used to binge on a popular fried chicken brand. His job meant he was on the motorway every day, so whenever he saw a service station and was hungry, he would crave fast food. He would eat it and then, within an hour, feel terrible to the point that he once had to pull over and be sick. Yet he kept on doing it for years. Why?

We will come back to the monkey brain later. But for now, just be aware that it is there, respect and acknowledge it and understand that it can be powerful, needs to be controlled and is looking for ways to get what it wants quickly, based on impulse rather than logical 'thinking', whether that be seeking immediate pleasures or making us react with anger. The monkey brain really comes to the fore during our toddler and teenage years, but adults also succumb to it often.

Setting yourself up for success

Some people find the 'engage' part of my **IDEAL** framework the hardest, as it requires some real action, not just contemplation. The aim is to get things sorted in your environment, because this will make it much easier to change your behaviours. People often say to me they've 'bought the book' but 'haven't started it', or that they know what kind of exercise they're going to do, but haven't got round to doing any yet. So make it easy for yourself.

'Engaging' basically means taking the first step in committing to actually doing what you have decided to do. And it feels so satisfying.

Preparing your environment is really important for creating good habits, but it's also vital when it comes to ditching bad ones.

The idea is to make it easy to start and repeat the good habit, and to make it really difficult to even think about the bad habit.

It's not about being hard on ourselves. To succeed, we need some perspective and self-compassion. Just look at the world around us. It generally encourages bad behaviours by making them too easy. It is too easy to make bad food choices; to stare at screens 24/7; to shop online any time we want; to binge on whatever we like, whenever we like, with no controls or regulation. And in these times of severe austerity, it is sometimes easier and cheaper to buy fried chicken and chips from the chicken shop for £2 than it is to cook a homemade meal. I have known older school children to do this up to three times a day.

But by changing our environments, we can exert some control over 'temptation', whether that's not having junk food in the house or keeping your smartphone locked away for one day a week. If you feel fear at the very *thought* of a day without your phone, that's OK – I did, too – but you really won't miss much, and you'll feel so much better without it that you'll actually look forward to not having your phone. And if everyone in your home does it at the same time, say, on a Sunday, then it makes it far more doable (this is a blend of 'Under orders' and 'Community spirit').

CHANGING THE BORING INTO SOMETHING FUN

I am going to dive into my own experiences here, to give you an idea of the kind of things I had to figure out when it came to tackling my own behaviours.

One of the things I realised from my wired and tired years as an off-duty junior doctor was that if you really want to, you can do things in bursts – and it's much easier if you also make them fun. Often, the job of a junior doctor is very much like that anyway – you work in adrenaline-fuelled surges of energy, so I wanted to use that skill to tackle chores that I found tiresome.

For instance, I used to get fed up with buying fruit and veg only for it to go off in the fridge after I'd had fast food three days on the trot. I also got frustrated by coming back to my digs to find a mountain of washing-up, with the sink full to the brim with dirty crockery and with no clean plates left to eat off.

I basically realised that if I could see humour or a challenge in something in a way that appealed to my monkey brain, then I could do it – however much I didn't fancy doing it. For me, that meant gamifying or making silly a really dull situation.

So, when it came to the washing-up, I would sing as I worked, aiming to see how long I could hold a phrase without taking a breath, and also to count how many items I could wash up within the length of that phrase. For ages, my go-to washing-up song was Whitney Houston's version of 'The Greatest Love of All', which contains some really long phrases. It sounds silly, but I never dreaded doing the washing-up after that.

For items about to go off in the fridge, I started making up random recipes to quickly use them up. I would pretend to be a makeshift doctor version of Jamie Oliver, performing a comedy voiceover to myself. I love doing impressions of celebs (admittedly not very well): 'Now, just look at those vegetables. Phwoaarr... Beau-i-ful... let's chuck that all in there with some extra virgin olive oil... mmm. Pukka!'

In reality, this ad-hoc cooking usually meant throwing together a combination of chillies, garlic, olive oil and any random green herbs, like parsley or coriander. Soy sauce and sesame oil usually featured, too. But what did it mean for me in reality? Well, occasionally, I would create a total howler of a dish that was a bit insipid, but the habit taught me that less is more when it comes to cooking with spices, and also that you can make really tasty healthy dishes out of the most random ingredients. Plus, of course, I reduced my food waste.

REPLACEMENTS

Frequently, I used to be tired after an on-call night, and that often meant I'd end up reaching for a beer or eating junk food for days on end (poor sleep makes our monkey brains come to the fore, as we crave comfort). I remember eating a whole packet of jam doughnuts one morning and feeling terrible afterwards. I do love a treat now and again, but it was happening far too often in that period of my life. Sometimes, the monkey brain has no 'off' switch, and so we need some other controls for this – namely replacements.

How does this work when it comes to our brains? If you've ever tried to take a smartphone away from a teenager who is busy on social media or watching videos, you will have seen that they react pretty badly. What you have briefly glimpsed is an example of an addiction-withdrawal behaviour.

Scrolling through social media feeds and getting 'likes' floods a part of the brain called the mesolimbic system (linked, once again, to the monkey brain) with dopamine, a chemical that is released when we experience pleasure. It naturally makes us crave more of that feeling if released excessively. The way to remove the phone with the least trauma is to replace the phone with something else that gives them some other form of lesser dopamine rush, like a hug, a hot drink or some praise.

It's not quite the same thing, but you can trick yourself into this when it comes to, say, reducing sugary foods. This can be made far easier if the sugary treat is replaced by something else. This option is great for people who struggle with going cold turkey – and I am no exception.

Years ago, in my old GP practice, we used to get given biscuits regularly by patients, and I would often munch my way through a whole pack by the end of a day. There's nothing wrong with the odd biscuit, but I was feeling sluggish and beginning to get bloated every day. This is really no different to Tom and his cigarettes in Egypt. I loved eating those deliciously crumbly Greek biscuits, but knew that a whole pack a day was no good for me! I didn't want to offend my patients, but I knew I had to get those biscuits out of my room or else I'd eat them, so I used to politely ask them to leave the biscuits behind the reception desk. The reception team would often give them away to local charities (this was before food banks existed). And in my room, I replaced the biscuits in the drawer with an apple and a bunch of berries each day or occasionally a banana. For the first two days, I really craved biscuits, but you know what? It passed. I started to feel lighter and brighter within a week. And that's how the **IDEAL** framework came about. I wanted to feel less sluggish; I realised it was the biscuits and that I needed to cut back; I decided I was going to do it; I made it easy by keeping them out of my room; I replaced them with something else; I felt better for it, and patted myself on the back for it. Boom: **IDEAL**.

I identified, defined, engaged, activated and looked back. Every day that I had fruit and not biscuits, I was so chuffed with myself. Not only that, but I started to feel better and more energetic quite quickly. This is also the method my motorway devouring patient used to get over his fried chicken cravings on the M1.

You've now taken the first step towards seeing how behaviour change works. You may have even started to imagine what you could change with the **IDEAL** framework, which we will revisit later.

It's great if you have, but to add more depth to this, we now need to look at the reasons *why* we make changes to benefit our health. It's time to move on from behaviours to biology.

CHAPTER SUMMARY

- Our behaviours are the keys to our health habits.

- Behaviour change is readily achievable if we make it easy.

- Use the IDEAL framework to get started.

- Be aware of your monkey brain, which can hijack good intentions thoughtlessly and on impulse.

8

SYSTEMS AND
SYMPTOMS

"*Symptom* – /ˈsɪm(p)təm/ – A physical or mental feature which is regarded as indicating a condition of disease..."

"*System* - /ˈsɪstəm/ – A set of things working together... or an interconnecting network; a complex whole."

Going back to how my health collapsed at forty, what I needed to understand was how my symptoms were connected to my biological systems. For me, that learning journey started over some beers a long time ago.

About twenty years ago, I was on my way to a friends' flat in central London. I got there to find he already had someone round: an old family friend of his who worked in finance.

The three of us chatted about all sorts before the friend started talking about how much he hated the way doctors just 'patch up' symptoms. I remember feeling quite annoyed, but not wishing to upset him, I nodded quietly as he said: 'For instance, if you have a runny nose or itchy skin, a doctor just gives you a spray or a cream, rather than finding out the actual reason behind the runny nose or the itchy skin...'

I recall thinking to myself that I could name several 'reasons' for a runny nose, including hay fever, sinusitis, allergies, infection with bacteria like *H. influenzae*, immune deficiency, overuse of decongestants and blood pressure tablets. I could reel off quite a few causes for itchy skin, such as eczema, psoriasis and scabies.

My view back then was that the nasal sprays and creams were pretty darn essential, depending on the cause. I had a real feeling of *l'esprit de l'escalier* once he'd left, and began to rattle off various arguments. I even said to my friend: 'He was a bit annoying, your mate, wasn't he?' I was a fairly typical overworked and defensive junior doctor back then.

But several months later, it dawned on me that what the clever finance guy was saying was he felt doctors seldom find the root cause of a symptom before they begin treating something, although the treatment might help and therefore be deemed effective. Sometimes we use what I call a 'seems reasonable' view, taking a Bayesian[15] probability-based approach ('common things are common') considering likelihoods and our best hunches. In a consultation, this often comes across as: 'Try this, and if it doesn't work, come back and we can try something else.' I'm sure that may sound familiar.

To be frank, there is a lot of 'What?' in medicine, but there isn't always as much 'Why?'. You can give the symptom of a runny nose a name like rhinitis; you can label erratic bowel habits as irritable bowel syndrome (IBS); and itching can be called pruritus to give it its medical name – but *why* is the person experiencing the symptom in the first place? Moreover, if you're not totally sure *why* they're having this symptom, then why give them a nasal spray for the runny nose, cream for the itchy skin or tablets for IBS if you don't *really* know what's caused it?

Of course I still prescribe medication regularly, but as soon as I understood where he was coming from, I couldn't stop thinking about it. And the more treatments I saw administered to people in hospital outpatients, the more I realised he had a point.

What he also got me thinking about is what I now understand to be *systems medicine*.[16] The human body is made up of several systems that are continuously communicating with each other. In the same way, we sometimes have symptoms that may all seem to be quite different, but are actually linked.

There are many systems in the body, but the main ones to consider are:

- the gastrointestinal system

- the immune system

- the endocrine system (hormones)

- the nervous system (brain)

- the cardiovascular system

- the musculoskeletal system

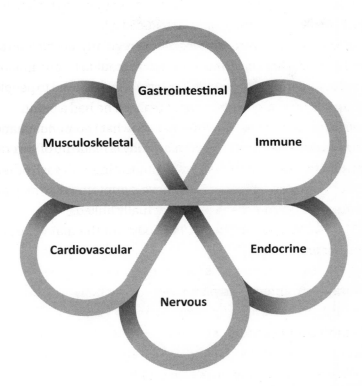

An easy way to imagine the interconnectedness of these systems is to think about what happens to your heart rate, the feeling in your gut, your breathing and your brain if you:

• unexpectedly drop a glass and it smashes

• have a terrible argument with a loved one

• suddenly receive some very bad news

• stay up all night revising for an exam on five cups of coffee

What I have just asked you to imagine is what happens when your systems malfunction temporarily. You experience *symptoms* (like a racing heart, butterflies in your tummy, feeling sad, emotional pain, a dry mouth, possibly a headache or muscle cramps). These are acute, short-lived examples, and we will come back to how this all relates to things like runny noses and itchy skin later, but for now just acknowledge that there is a link between *symptoms* and *systems*.

How systems relate to symptoms

In those stressful situations I mentioned above, you were able to imagine what could rapidly happen to your body systems. The same things, however, effectively happen in slow motion over many months or years. In essence, what we do and what happens to us have direct effects on our biological systems.

Eating, moving, sleeping, dealing with stress, changes in our environment, how much we get outdoors, our relationships, our homes – all of these things affect our biological systems.

> To put it quite simply, if our **systems** are out of whack, then we may start to experience **symptoms**. But if we change our **behaviours**, this can change how our systems work, thereby resolving our symptoms.

What gives rise to symptoms	*Systems involved*
Diet	Gastrointestinal
Exercise	Immune
Stress	Endocrine
Sleep	Nervous
Environment	Cardiovascular
Genetics	Musculoskeletal
Past infections	
Sunlight	

Many of you will have experienced this. Something in your routine changes, and your symptoms change as a result. Just like my happy accident with not drinking coffee made me feel less tired and edgy. Every week in my surgery, I hear stories like, 'I used to get really bad heartburn in my twenties, but it went away once I moved home and started cooking more,' or, 'My back pain used to be terrible, until I changed my mattress last year.' These are, of course, quite straightforward examples.

Now, when I talk about symptoms, I must stress that I'm not talking about 'acute' medical symptoms (things that happen suddenly), like strokes, heart attacks or infections that need urgent treatment (although some of these, too, are often effectively an end result of a type of 'system malfunction'). Instead, I am referring more to symptoms that descend on us gradually, such as fatigue, persistent heartburn, anxiety, unexplained headaches, stress, insomnia, low mood, poor skin, persistent tummy aches, joint pains, recurrent illness and hard-to-manage long-term conditions that can significantly affect our day-to-day quality of life. And the additional rub is that some of these symptoms can be an early warning sign or harbinger of a future long-term condition.

How things go wrong: the water leak

Forgetting the body for a minute, let us think about the systems that make a home function, such as plumbing, drainage, electrical, heating, Wi-Fi and alarm systems. There is a lot of overlap between these systems which all provide a service. For your home to function properly, all of them need to be working well at the same time.

For a real-life example of system malfunction, let's imagine the dreaded bathroom leak. It might be upstairs, or in your neighbour's flat above yours. It starts to show as a brown patch on your ceiling (this is the first symptom, if you like), and before you know it, it's leaked into the living room light switch, causing a random power cut. The leak then creates a damp wall, leading to a mould problem that gradually destroys the plaster and the timber under the floor. Wet rot then sets in, and the house is now in need of urgent attention. The point is that a seemingly innocuous leak from a bath or shower can cause utter havoc over time. And painting over the new brown patch on the ceiling is never a realistic long-term option.

It's exactly the same principle with our bodies. If one system starts to go wrong, then slowly but surely, others will, too, until we find and fix the metaphorical 'leak'.

While I prescribe medication regularly, and sometimes it may be the best solution, one way of looking at the aim in the longer term is to try to intervene at the stage of system malfunction before it develops into an actual condition or disease. As we have just seen, the first warning sign for system malfunction is often a symptom.

How do we find out what's wrong?

THE HEALTH LOOP

It's time for me to introduce you to the **Health Loop**. This is the first part of your *Health Fix* toolkit. It's firmly based on my Symptom Web®, which is something I use in teaching, but the principles are identical. In my view, the eight factors that make up this 'loop' have the biggest impact on our health on a day-to-day basis. They give rise to symptoms, but they are also the factors that affect our biological systems in the long term. Quite simply, the **Health Loop** turns *what* into *why*.

This is the starting point for laying out the reason for our symptoms and how we can work out which systems might not be working optimally.

Think of the **Health Loop** as your own equivalent of artificial intelligence (AI) – natural intelligence (or NI), if you like. It's a way of translating what your body is telling you by looking at logical clues. To be clear, this is not an algorithm and it is not automation. It's based on facts. It is based purely on the story of you and your health. It just helps bring all of it into sharp focus. If you're a fan of precision medicine and you can afford all the gizmos that give you data, then great – this will work well with that, but it is designed to be accessible to all.

Once you are able to look at your own **Health Loop** and get a handle on your habits, you will be able to tweak and modify what you do in order to improve your health. As you will see, it is not just about diet and exercise.

Your symptoms can be almost any that have crept up on you over a period of time. Common ones I see in practice include anxiety, pain and fatigue, or they could be related to a long-term condition, such as depression, eczema, type 2 diabetes, high blood pressure, IBS or dermatitis.

The eight elements of the **Health Loop** are pretty self-explanatory, but for avoidance of doubt, let's go through them. First, take a look at it for a minute or so. Have a good stare at it.

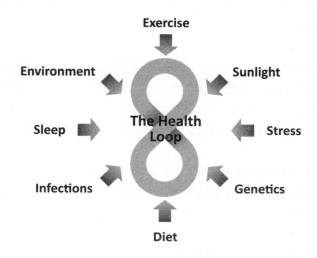

You will see real-life examples in the next section of the book, but here is a summary:

Exercise – This is to do with posture, movement and your levels of physical activity, which we know are important for all-round good health. Exercise increases blood flow via nitric oxide and is beneficial for every system in the body.

Sunlight – This is about your exposure to sunlight and the impact on your vitamin D levels, which are involved in many important functions.

Genetics – This, in essence, is your family history of any medical conditions that might be relevant to your own health. There are also certain genes that are specific to certain conditions. Of course we cannot change our genes but we can change how they are 'expressed'.

Stress – What are your stress levels like? Stress is a well-known contributory factor to illness across the board (including depression, skin conditions, high blood pressure, digestive problems and autoimmune diseases).[17]

Diet – Food is to be enjoyed, but also acts as 'information' for your immune system by the time it is digested. How, what and when we eat are important.

Infections – This is about infections you may have had in the past (such as gastroenteritis, recurrent tonsillitis, flu, COVID or glandular fever), as they can have an effect on your immune system for years down the line. We tend to forget about them once we recover.

Sleep – Sleep is a key factor in health, and good-quality sleep can help to prevent many long-term conditions.[18]

Environment – Are you in a toxic relationship? Do you have mould in your home? Are you struggling with finances or your living arrangements? Do you have a bully for a boss? Are you lacking purpose in your life? Environment encompasses all of these and more.

The systems

Going back to my rather simple analogy of the house and the water leak as a symptom that can then affect other home systems, it's time to look at our own biological systems and what they do for us as their main functions.

You will notice when looking at the systems on the opposite page that certain functions, like sleep and nutrients, appear in more than one system. These systems overlap – and this is a key point here. No one system can work alone. Even the leaky shower needs electricity for its pump, as well as plumbing and a water supply. But this interconnectedness also works the other way. One intervention can hit many bases when it comes to our biological systems.

The nervous system (brain)
Responsible for:
- mood
- memory
- concentration
- imagination
- thinking
- personality
- speech
- sleep
- the control of movement and organs
- the control of breathing
- sensation
- balance

The musculoskeletal system
Responsible for:
- enabling movement, strength and balance
- protecting organs
- storing minerals
- making blood cells

The gastrointestinal system (gut)
Responsible for:
- digestion
- the absorption of nutrients
- nourishing our immune system

The immune system
Responsible for:
- protecting us from illness with an appropriate immune response

The endocrine system (hormones)
Responsible for:
- growth
- the metabolism of nutrients
- sexual function
- appetite
- sleep
- mood

The cardiovascular system
Responsible for:
- controlling blood pressure
- controlling heart rate
- providing blood and oxygen to organs
- clotting wounds

A good example is the multiple benefits of exercise. If we look at the benefits of exercise at a slightly deeper level than just accepting that it is 'good for us', just a few of its systemic benefits to our biology include:

- an increase in nitric oxide, leading to improved blood flow (cardiovascular system)

• an increase in a protein called BDNF (brain-derived neuro-trophic factor) in the brain, which prevents Alzheimer's disease (nervous system)

• a reduction in insulin resistance (endocrine system) which can mean a reduced risk of developing type 2 diabetes

Nerves, blood vessels, hormones and mucosal tissue (the inner linings of our body) may all be separate entities, but they are dependent on each other providing gateways between different systems. And exercise is just one type of lifestyle activity that touches all of these bases.

This interconnectedness is not surprising, as there is so much going on in our bodies twenty-four hours a day, in terms of biochemistry and physiology, simply to keep us alive. This crucial interplay between systems is also part of the reason why changing simple things can improve our overall health so much.

One change can bestow multiple benefits. And this method will allow you to hone in on what the quick wins might be.

The Lifestyle Prescription

A Lifestyle Prescription is simply a set of agreed actions that a patient and practitioner come up with together, but in the case of *The Health Fix*, you will learn how to generate your own. This is a great starting point for change, as it involves laying out some simple strategies. Some people find the word 'lifestyle' a bit grating, especially when we talk about 'lifestyle medicine'.[19] I actually co-author, write and teach a course called 'Prescribing Lifestyle Medicine'. Ironically, I myself do not like the term. The truth is, though, there isn't really a better word than 'lifestyle' to describe what it really means. No definition is perfect, but for the context of this book, I would like you to think of the word 'lifestyle' as having either of these definitions:

LIFESTYLE = HABITS + LUCK
or
LIFESTYLE = BEHAVIOURS + ENVIRONMENT

THINK ABOUT YOUR TYPICAL DAY

In my own clinical practice, once I have listened carefully to someone's symptoms, including how these symptoms started and how long they have been going on, the next thing I will do is ask the patient to tell me about their typical day. This gives me so much useful information about them; it's almost like a snapshot of their life as it currently is.

I have their medical history in front of me on my screen (you should know most of your own medical history, and if you do not, then please try to find out). In addition to that, the account of their typical day will give me much of the information I need to start filling in their **Health Loop** in my head.

What we are trying to do is to match up **lifestyle** with **symptoms**, and **symptoms** with **systems**.

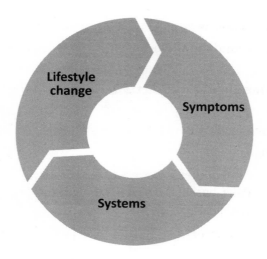

Once you are armed with your own medical history, your own typical day and the **Health Loop**, you have everything you need to examine in order to reach the destination of a **Lifestyle Prescription**. Here's an example of the kind of thing a doctor might routinely hear in the consulting room or on the phone...

Matt is a thirty-eight-year-old property renovations manager. He lives alone, but has loads of good mates locally. Matt has multiple symptoms.

In terms of his medical history, his dad has type 2 diabetes and Matt himself had his appendix out at the age of thirteen, and his tonsils out at eighteen. He's not on any medication at the moment.

Here is Matt's typical day:

- He wakes up at 7am, feeling very tired – he has to force himself out of bed.

- He eats a bowl of cereal and has a cup of tea while quickly pacing around the kitchen.

- He showers and quickly brushes his teeth.

- He drives to work by 9am in heavy traffic (he's always rushing).

- He has a desk-based office job with some site visits now and again. Work is stressful, and he's busy working non-stop from 9am to 1pm.

- He has a sandwich at 1pm with a fizzy drink and an apple (he 'hoofs it down on the go', to use his own words).

- He then works solidly from 2–6pm, with some tea and biscuits to keep going.

- He drives back home, feeling tired. About once a week, he stops at the gym to use the treadmill, but feels exhausted afterwards.

- At 7pm, he flops on the sofa to watch TV.

- He has dinner at 8pm – usually pasta, stir-fry or sausage and chips, with one or two beers, or a few more at weekends.

- At 9pm, he finishes off his work emails.

- By 10pm, he'll be dozing on the sofa in front of the TV, chatting on WhatsApp and having snacks like crisps and biscuits.

- He sleeps poorly, with his sleep usually broken, and he often watches box sets at night in bed.

Matt's story is fairly typical. In the next chapter, we will take a closer look at stories like Matt's and the power of applying the **Health Loop** to create behaviour change.

The Health Fix toolkit

The Health Fix toolkit consists of:
- your typical day

- your medical history

- your **Health Loop**

- your **Lifestyle Prescription**

Sitting alongside this are:
- the **IDEAL** framework

- '**How, what and when**' (we will explore this shortly)

- Acknowledging and managing your monkey brain

As we go through the case studies and stories in the coming chapters, this process will become clearer. Think of it as an infinite loop which can be repeated if necessary.

CHAPTER SUMMARY

- Changing your behaviours is key to improving your health.

- These changes will have an impact on your biological systems.

- Your biological systems are linked to your symptoms.

- Think about your typical day and your medical history.

- The **Health Loop** will lay out why you are experiencing symptoms and gives you a starting point from which you can work towards a **Lifestyle Prescription**.

II

THE ASPIRATIONS

"The wish for healing has always been half of health."
Seneca

Case studies

I am hoping that the importance of our behaviour, our biology and the fact that symptoms and systems are linked is now clear in your mind. It's now time to look at some real-world examples.

Most of us would agree that health really is wealth, but our time on earth is finite and short, so we want to enjoy it! I have seen so many patients over the years who have had problems that have driven them to despair in terms of their quality of life. Most people want the same thing: to feel better. Each of us has our own unique story and health aspirations, but most of us want a long and healthy life, full of vitality, free of pain and illness.

Each case you are about to read has one major theme reflected in its title as the person's main health wish or aspiration. You will see there is a lot of overlap, and often more than one symptom is involved. You will get to see each person's **Health Loop** laid out, and get a good feel for them as individuals, and we will then explore the process of how their **Lifestyle Prescription** was generated and the effect it had on them. Finally, we will also dip in and out of the science and evidence to understand why these changes worked as we go through each case. It is important to 'get under the bonnet' in this way, in order to get to the *why* and not just focus on the *what*.

Occasionally, you will find a **Deep Dive** section, which examines more closely the science related to the case. Feel free to skip these if you prefer to read them later. The cases are presented in no particular order. I hope they will give you an insight into what is happening around us all the time. First, I am going to introduce you to Amelia, who craved one main thing as her health wish: to have more energy.

8

'I WANT MORE ENERGY'

'I'm just tired all the time, doctor...' Commonly referred to as 'TATT' by medics (short for 'tired all the time'), around ten to 18% of people in the UK report tiredness.[20] One of the most common 'soft' medical wishes we doctors hear is, 'I just wish I had more energy.'

There are several medical reasons for tiredness and fatigue. If you have tried all the basics and drawn a blank, then you may wish to discuss it with your healthcare provider to rule out the following (not exhaustive) list:[21]

- high blood pressure

- anaemia

- an underactive thyroid

- type 2 diabetes

- vitamin D and/or vitamin B12 deficiency

- coeliac disease or other autoimmune conditions

- Lyme disease

- long COVID

- glandular fever (caused by the Epstein-Barr virus)

Blood pressure can be checked at home these days with an auto-mated cuff from a supermarket or pharmacy, or many healthcare providers will check it for you. Most of the other items on the list can be ruled out by blood tests. Blood tests can be useful, particularly if you have a family history of anything on the list (remember that genetics and your family history make up part of your **Health Loop**). More often than not, though, blood tests for tiredness come back 'normal'.

Meet Amelia. She was a healthy nineteen-year-old who had 'never had a day of illness in her life', according to her dad, who came with her to see me, but for quite a while she had been feeling tired all the time and was told by a doctor that she most likely had chronic fatigue.

Amelia told me she had stopped being able to play hockey, for which she was university captain. She had also been falling asleep by 8pm and struggling to get out of bed in the mornings for the last six months. She was clearly a sporty type, as her dad reeled off the number of trophies she had won, but because she wasn't feeling particularly well, this sportiness wasn't obvious in the consultation. No one is at their best when they feel unwell, and as a doctor, I am only too mindful of this.

Amelia told me how she had developed daily tummy aches and seemed to suddenly have brittle nails, but her main complaint was overwhelming tiredness: 'I could just stay in bed all day. I feel like I've got no energy. I can't do anything. After five minutes of hockey training, I'm just exhausted.' Her coursework was also beginning to suffer, and she had big exams coming up. She looked really down, and was frankly desperate.

After several minutes of saying she had never been ill, and a bit more drilling down on the events of the past year, she revealed that she had broken up with her long-term boyfriend and fallen out with a university friend. Although not related, both incidents had taken place just over eight months before. These were both hugely stressful events. She had then had two urine infections back to back, which required treatment with antibiotics.

Amelia had already seen several doctors about her tiredness. They had carried out a full panel of blood tests that came back normal, including a test for coeliac disease and vitamin D and vitamin B12 levels. They put her symptoms down to a virus (this was before COVID), mild depression, or unexplained fatigue, and she was becoming more frustrated as there was lots of conjecture but no answers. For me, it was case closed as soon as I got the whole story. I am going to take you through what happened to Amelia, step by step, and how we came up with a **Lifestyle Prescription** for her.

Once I'd established there was nothing else of note in her medical history, I asked Amelia to tell me about her typical day:

- She wakes up tired at 7.30am.

- For breakfast, she eats a popular wheat-based cereal with milk, or toast and tea.

- At 8.30am, her university day begins. She is already tired and bloated, and begins to get a tummy ache.

- At 11am, she takes a break and eats a granola bar.

- She has lunch at 1pm: a sandwich and crisps plus fizzy water.

- At 4pm, she finishes uni classes (feeling very tired by now).

- At 5pm, she goes to hockey practice, but quickly feels exhausted and leaves.

- She has dinner at 6.30pm: pasta, rice or chicken.

- At 7pm, she will be on her phone, at her computer doing coursework, or reading a book.

- By 8pm she will be exhausted, and she'll be in bed by 9pm at the latest, often with some snacks. Often wakes up thirsty at night.

- She sleeps poorly at night and feels restless, with a painful, bloated tummy.

Apart from her symptoms of bloating and tiredness, for me the thing that really stuck out was that her diet was not varied, and contained hardly any fruit or veg. So this was a start in itself, but probably didn't explain why Amelia was quite so overwhelmingly tired. So let's start by filling in Amelia's **Health Loop**.

Amelia's Health Loop

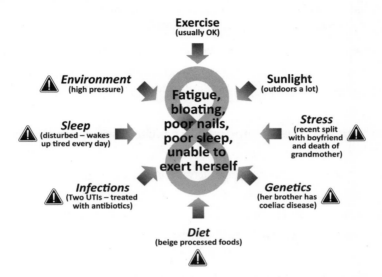

Immediately, we can clearly see that her **diet** and **sleep** are both issues that need addressing. We can come back to these. Next, we simply work around the rest of the remaining **Health Loop** factors to see what is relevant.

Exercise – Amelia had been previously fit and active, but was now struggling to hit her usual levels of fitness because of her exhaustion.

Sunlight – Amelia certainly seemed to get outdoors a lot, and so I wasn't too worried about her sunlight exposure. Her blood tests showed her vitamin D levels were normal.

Stress – Stress affects us in many ways,[22] as many of us will have experienced, but one impact it has is that it increases a hormone called cortisol, which affects blood pressure, sleep, concentration and energy. It also affects our immune system and its responses. Amelia had been through two stressful life events, but also had current stress from not being able to play sport and the thought of her impending exams.

Genetics – Amelia's brother has coeliac disease, which is an allergy to gluten, a group of proteins found in wheat (see **Deep Dive** on page 69 for more information).

Infections – Amelia had had two urine infections eight months before, both requiring antibiotics.

Environment – Amelia had a supportive home environment, but it's possible there was quite a lot of pressure around sport and university exams.

Amelia had gone from being a healthy teenager to someone who was struggling to get out of bed. Her timeline shows us what happened – and when. A combination of stress, infections, poor diet and pressure had triggered her low mood and symptoms of bloating and fatigue. But why was it happening now? And how? How could a healthy person slowly become ill over a few months with nothing showing up on tests? It is easy to forget that illness can be cumulative, and a timeline really helps us visualise this. One thing happens, then another, then another – and eventually, it can all add up and can bring a person to a tipping point. Health and illness are often about thresholds.

Sometimes it can be helpful to draw a story out on a timeline:

Amelia's timeline

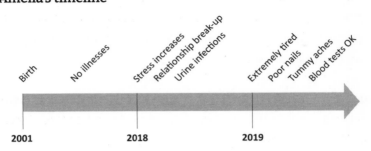

Stress, infections and antibiotics – and their effect on the gut and immune system

Looking at her **Health Loop**, it's clear to see that Amelia had experienced stress and infections, which had acted as a quick double-hit to her immune system.

We have talked a little about stress, but receiving treatment for simple infections, such as urine infections and tonsillitis, can also have a negative effect on the immune system.

Each time we take a course of antibiotics for these kinds of infections (and antibiotics may be entirely necessary), they have a negative effect on the immune system. This is because antibiotics cannot tell the difference between good and bad bacteria, so they effectively wipe out both, getting rid of the bad bacteria causing the infection, but also almost all of the good bacteria in the gut (known as gut flora or the microbiome). This good bacteria can be wiped out for anything from a few weeks to up to a year each time we take antibiotics.[23] This disruption of the microbiome, although often temporary, can have myriad effects on us, including tiredness, diarrhoea, bloating, and even low mood. I see this almost every single week in my NHS practice, and you may have experienced the same thing yourself.

Approximately 70% of the immune system is found in the inner lining of the gut wall, and 'good' bacteria is essentially responsible for 'feeding' the immune system, allowing it to function appropriately. We can think of the gut as an entry point into the immune system.[24] Bearing in mind it protects us from illness, keeping our gut flora in a good state is key to our immune function.

Amelia had background issues as well as her stress and antibiotic use. These were revealed by her typical day. Her diet was quite 'beige' and low in nutrients: bread, cakes, biscuits, pasta, cereal; all tasty, but lacking the nutrients needed to really nourish the gut. Her already poor flora (from the antibiotics) coupled with her sub-optimal diet, had married up to give her new symptoms of bloating after meals and tummy aches. She had managed to get by on her current diet for years, probably because of her generally healthy constitution, but these recent events had tipped the balance and her body was no longer coping with it. Once you put all of these factors into the mix, it's pretty obvious why Amelia's health collapsed. And these issues were affecting both her brain and her body. Remember: systems are linked to symptoms.

> **Amelia:**
> (Poor diet + stress + infection + antibiotics) = fatigue, brittle nails, bloating, low mood

So, with this in mind, we essentially needed to somehow reverse the effects of all of the stand-out sections in her **Health Loop**. How? Well, in order to help her get better, we first needed to look more closely at her habits. The idea is to come up with a plan based on changing not just *what* she does, but *how* and *when* she does it. This is really important. Amelia was very motivated to change her habits as she was so desperate to feel better, so there was no need for any kind of **IDEAL** framework here.

How, what and when?

The first thing to remind ourselves about from **The Foundations** section of this book is that symptoms are often linked to systems 'going wrong'. To recap, Amelia's beige diet probably hadn't been affecting her a year ago, but it was now almost certainly an issue. Her gut had since been affected by both antibiotics and stress.[25] As mentioned earlier, this can have a negative effect on gut bacteria and can manifest as bloating after meals. It also makes it harder to absorb any nutrients available, as the lining of the gut is often slightly inflamed because of the shift towards poorer gut flora. Amelia's poor nail health was almost certainly a sign of micronutrient deficiency (iron, zinc and magnesium).[26]

We need to look at each **Health Loop** area in turn when laying out someone's story, but when it comes to their habits, we usually need to explore a bit further and ask three simple questions. The answers will not only help us complete the **Health Loop** and understand their medical history, but will also inform their **Lifestyle Prescription**. These simple questions are:

How?

What?

When?

How does Amelia eat? *What* does she eat? *When* does she eat? Let's stop and have a think about this. The questions may not always work in terms of syntax, but the same principles apply to sleep, movement and rest. We can't apply them to everything we do, but **How, What and When** work well for most of our daily activities. Changing the **How, What and When** can totally change how we feel.

Amelia agreed to reduce – and, if possible, remove – her excess of beige foods and replace them with a better diet. She would incorporate more chicken, fish, fruits, vegetables and nuts (often called whole foods as they are not processed), rather than relying on just cereals, sandwiches, biscuits and pasta. Beige foods may be tasty and filling, but teenagers often become iron-deficient because these foods are not high in nutrients, whereas whole foods, like nuts, fruits and vegetables, are nutrient packed. Processed and highly processed foods (e.g. instant noodles or tinned hot dog sausages) are food that are not in their natural state and, as such, are prone to eliciting abnormal reactions from our immune systems.[27]

Next, regarding Amelia's stress levels, which I felt were still high, I could see that based on her 'typical day', she was never really switching off, so I asked her to 'do nothing' for up to five minutes a day, each day. She was willing to try this and incorporate proper 'down time' into her days, with relaxing breathing exercises such as belly breathing, which you will read about on page 178. These breathing exercises have a rapid calming effect on the nervous system via the vagus nerve (an important nerve linking the brain to the gut). The more this kind of practice is repeated, the greater the benefits. Most people who try this kind of practice feel so much better after two weeks or so, and some actually get addicted to doing it. And *voilà* – you have a new healthy habit.

My one-minute recharge

As I pointed out at the beginning of the book, my own health had declined in 2014. One of my **Health Loop** triggers was stress. Something I do to this day is what I call a one-minute recharge. I sit in the car when I get to work and breathe slowly – sometimes I breathe in for a count of five, hold for five, then breathe out for seven – but usually I just do some slow, deep breathing. Within a minute, I am set for the day, I feel calmer and am much less likely to feel stress, even when faced with it. I do the same when I get home. I sit in the car for a minute to 'leave my doctor's bag' at the front door before entering the house. Just spending these two indulgent minutes a day can help activate your vagus nerve, bringing on a swathe of calm. If you can't do five minutes, just do one.[28]

As for infections, there was a need to replenish Amelia's gut flora to support her immune system. Over time, this is best done with 'prebiotic' foods, such as bananas, berries and green vegetables, as they nourish the gut over a long period to help create healthy populations of bacteria that support the immune system.[29] Chatting to Amelia, we agreed the easiest foods for her to incorporate would be bananas, apples and peas. She had also forgotten how much she loved cherries, which are full of fibre and nutrients. It is worth noting that sometimes prebiotic foods themselves cause bloating, particularly if the gut flora is not in a good state.

A quicker way to replenish gut bacteria is to take a probiotic supplement for a month, which Amelia's dad bought for her from a local chemist. Probiotics flood the gut with beneficial bacteria to restore what has been wiped out by antibiotics. So, Amelia's **Lifestyle Prescription** had been agreed. I scribbled it on a sticky note:

- Drink more water.

- Eat less beige processed food, and adopt a more whole-food-based diet with fruit and veg. Eat more slowly, and avoid snacking before bed.

- Spend five minutes doing 'nothing' or breathing exercises each day.

- Take a probiotic called LGG®.[30]

Deep Dive: Coeliac disease

The eagle-eyed among you will have noted that Amelia's brother has coeliac disease. Is this relevant? The answer is – possibly. Coeliac disease is an allergy to gluten, a protein found in wheat. This means food likes pasta, wheat-based cereals, cakes, pizza, biscuits, soy sauce, taramasalata and a whole host of other foods are off the menu, as they cause an immune response in the form of antibodies to gluten.

Despite Amelia testing negative for coeliac disease (which tests for whether she is making antibodies to gluten), she may well carry a genetic marker that is linked to it, because she has a first-degree relative with the condition. Science tells us our genes are sections of our DNA which are related to a particular function. Genes are arranged along our twenty-three pairs of chromosomes which are inherited from each of our parents.

Almost everyone with coeliac disease (99%) has one of two specific genetic subtypes, called HLA DQ2 or HLA DQ8.[31] These HLAs are clusters of genes on chromosome 6 that essentially 'code' for surface proteins on our cells. HLAs are responsible for regulating our immune system. In coeliac disease, it is these cellular surface proteins, found in the small intestine of the gut, that interact with gluten, leading to a sequence of events that result in an 'antibody response' which causes symptoms such as abdominal pain, diarrhoea and more. Coeliac disease is an example of an autoimmune disease where the immune system is triggered to attack the body's own tissues but specifically it happens in people with HLAs DQ2 or DQ8.

Although Amelia tested negative for the antibodies in coeliac disease, this simply means she was not making antibodies to gluten at that moment in time. But if she has either the HLA DQ2 or DQ8 gene subtypes, then the more gluten she consumes, there is a 10–20% likelihood that she may go on to develop the condition during her life through repeated exposure to gluten. This is a really good example of genetics loading the gun (the HLAs) and our environment pulling the trigger (gluten). You cannot change your genes, but you can change the way they are expressed, depending on your habits. When Amelia changed her diet, she stopped consuming almost all wheat products, and therefore gluten. This was actually by accident, as she was simply avoiding beige foods, but this seemed to help her symptoms greatly.

In my clinical practice, if someone has a family member with coeliac disease and keeps getting gut symptoms after eating gluten-containing products, but tests negative on a coeliac blood test, I tell them they may wish to have a genetic test for HLA DQ2 and DQ8 privately (if they have the means). DNA testing is unfortunately not routinely available in the NHS.

A negative result (if neither HLA subtype is found) practically excludes coeliac disease, as almost 99% of people with it have one or both of the two HLA subtypes. A positive result simply means the person is in the 40% of the population with these HLA subtypes, and that coeliac disease may develop in future if they continue to eat gluten.

After just six weeks of following her **Lifestyle Prescription**, Amelia was feeling much better. She felt she had aced her year-end exams and was back to playing top-level hockey with her university team. Her mood was back to normal, her energy was restored, and she was feeling like her old self again.

Together, we had put the pieces of a puzzle together based on her unique story to find a solution that would work for her.

The Drawstring Effect

Amelia's case beautifully demonstrates the interplay of systems in medicine: once you fix one issue, other things start to fix themselves.

The **Health Loop** lays everything out. Once you start gently 'pulling' on the obvious parts of the loop to tighten things up, your whole system improves and becomes more efficient.

For instance, a better diet may lead to better mood or better sleep, not just a less bloated stomach. As our biological systems are all interconnected, by gently doing several things at once, you can quickly improve your whole system – which is exactly what Amelia did.

The same happens with habits. Here is an example:

You start to go to bed earlier.

This makes you less irritable in the morning.

As a result, you are nicer to your family in the mornings...

... which means you feel happier during your workday...

... and so you eat less comfort or junk food...

... and come home feeling less tired.

This is what I call the **Drawstring Effect**, and it is truly wonderful to experience. You will see this again and again in the case studies that follow, and hopefully in your own life. In Amelia's case, it was her swift change in what and when she ate, plus the addition of relaxation, that seemed to be the tighteners in her **Health Loop**, allowing her whole system to function better, thereby resolving many of her symptoms.

CHAPTER SUMMARY

- Tiredness and fatigue can have undiagnosed medical causes.

- Our energy levels can be affected by insults to the immune system, such as stress or antibiotics.

- High-nutrient foods nourish the gut and immune system.

- Simple changes can have knock-on effects quickly – remember the **Drawstring Effect**.

8

'I WANT BETTER DIGESTION'

When I was at medical school in the early 1990s, I remember having a 'putting the world to rights' conversation with some mates in our local pub, The Distillers in Hammersmith. We were trying to predict the future in terms of which medical specialties would be the busiest in our working lives. One of my friends was adamant it would be respiratory medicine, because of worsening air pollution; another said gastroenterology, because of the rise in cheap supermarket beer, alcopops and fast food (all of which, ironically, we often lived on back then, as 'invincible' students). I remember saying it would be general practice that took the biggest toll, because it would be harder to see hospital specialists as more work got pushed into the community. We were all correct, in a way. All of those disciplines are far busier now according to data from NHS Digital and NHS England. Come to think of it, not a day goes by in my clinical practice when someone doesn't consult me about respiratory or gut symptoms.

Let me introduce Gary. Now, before you read on, I will tell you at this point that his is a 'gut story'. He's a hairdresser who'd had ten years of heartburn, with two normal endoscopy tests and no sign of infection with *H. pylori* (a bacterium that can cause intractable heartburn symptoms). He was on maximum acid-blocking medication, but was still getting heartburn every single day. He had tried to cut out spicy foods and alcohol, but it made no difference and he was often waking in the night with heartburn.

Gary's typical day was interesting. He would get up at around 7.30am and walk to work, which took about twenty minutes, picking up a latte and a croissant or muffin to eat on the way. He runs a salon with his business partner, so is on his feet all day – it's busy. Gary would grab tea and biscuits and a sandwich on the go. Work was quite stressful, he told me. They have an extra stylist on a Saturday, but in the week it's just the two of them.

In the evenings, Gary might pop to the gym on the way home, but once he was home, he would usually hit the sofa, often falling asleep there. His favourite dinners were usually pasta, curries or roast chicken. He drank alcohol rarely; if he did drink, it was only at weekends.

Looking at Gary's medical history, I could see he had suffered with recurrent ear infections for many years as a child, and ultimately had to have surgery on his eardrum. Gary was fit and went to the gym twice a week. I noticed during our examination that he had good muscle tone and there was no abdominal abnormality detected but he had brittle nails.

There were a few things that jumped out at me when it came to Gary's **Health Loop**, based on his medical history and his typical day. Let's take a look at them.

Gary's Health Loop

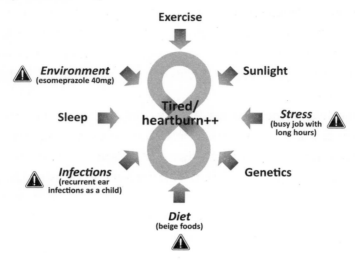

Let's think about what comes next. Gary's typical day gives us a number of clues. Let's look at what it tells us about his **How, What and When**.

Gary's typical day was interesting. He would get up at around 7.30am and **walk to work,** *which took about twenty minutes,* **picking up a latte and a croissant or muffin to eat on the way**. *He runs a salon with his business partner, so is* **on his feet all day** *– it's busy. Gary would grab* **tea and biscuits and a sandwich on the go**. **Work was quite stressful,** *he told me. They have an extra stylist on a Saturday, but in the week it's just the two of them.*

The first thing that hit me was that when it came to eating, Gary needed to make some major changes. During the day, he was eating all his meals while walking and standing. The **How, What and When** of his eating was not ideal, to say the least.

Gary's food intake during the day was rushed and low in nutrients (rather like Amelia's was). He was eating food that is harder to digest than whole foods, and he was eating it while standing or on the go. Standing while eating means that your digestive enzymes (which break down food) do not get ample time to work.[32] An enzyme in the mouth called salivary amylase starts the process of breaking down carbohydrate foods, but if you eat quickly or do not chew your food enough, this vital step is missed out before further enzymes released from the pancreas kick in later in the digestive process.

This was a triple hit for Gary:

- He was eating food that's hard to digest.

- He was eating standing up, which requires more digestive power.

- He was eating quickly.

I had also sent Gary for some blood tests as he was so tired, and they showed low levels for vitamin D and vitamin B12 – he wasn't deficient, but almost. The latter was possibly to do with his medication; acid-suppressing drugs (called proton-pump inhibitors) taken over many years can lead to a lack of absorption of certain vitamins and minerals.[33]

Looking at the rest of his **Health Loop**, the main issues were his high workload, which was causing him stress, and his childhood ear infections and the resulting numerous courses of antibiotics. As with Amelia, this element of Gary's story pointed towards poor gut flora, which needed addressing. The timeline was different, though. Gary had taken a lot of antibiotics for a few years a long time ago.

This was the **Lifestyle Prescription** that Gary and I agreed upon.

- Eat more whole foods, especially fish and vegetables. Eat slowly, chew properly and sit down to eat. Eat dinner earlier, as eating late makes digestion even harder.

- Buy less junk food and have more whole foods to snack on (carrot sticks, apples, etc.).

- Keep up good levels of movement, but no eating on the go.

- Take a probiotic supplement, and vitamin D and B12 sprays.

What happened over the next few weeks seemed astonishing to Gary, but now that you can see the 'working' behind the changes he made, perhaps you will not be quite so surprised.

Within two weeks, he was feeling almost no heartburn symptoms. Within four weeks, he had been able to halve his medication, and within six weeks, he had stopped it altogether – and also felt a lot more energetic.

Gary was really focused, as he was so desperate to get better, so he had no difficulty in activating or engaging with these changes. He didn't need to hold the **IDEAL** framework in his head.

Also, remember the power of marginal gains (see page 28)

and that powerful **Drawstring Effect**? These were certainly at play with Gary. Although Gary's story was a gut story, and Amelia's was a 'tiredness' story, there are a few similarities between them. This is simply because of the relationship between systems and symptoms.

Deep Dive: The gut as a system and its link to autoimmunity

I wanted to add this section, as I think it is important to explain the gut and the microbiome, and why diet can be so important. During the course of this book, you will see that I tend to play down diet a bit, and that's because it's not actually always one of the strings that needs pulling on. But if you think about it, almost all of us eat each day, and therefore the digestive system is one of the more important systems governing our health, arguably second only to the brain and nervous system.

It's important to explain why. When we think about Amelia, for example, she was beginning to get symptoms affecting her whole body. There were a few reasons for this, but one of them was that she was almost certainly well on the way to developing SIBO (small intestinal bacterial overgrowth).[34] In basic terms, SIBO is when harmful or rare gut bacteria outnumber beneficial ones. This can cause immediate bloating after meals (a hallmark symptom) or IBS-type symptoms. SIBO often presents with immediate bloating after meals, has to be detected via breath testing

---

before it can be treated appropriately.

One of the issues with SIBO (or 'blind loop syndrome', as it was taught at medical school) is that it coexists with so many symptoms beyond the gut, including rashes, fatigue, joint and muscle pains, and sometimes fever. Why? How does it even do that? I never got an explanation at medical school. Well, the first thing is that many things can help lead to the development of SIBO, including the overuse of antibiotics, smoking, stress, poor gall bladder function and low stomach acid. But how exactly does a problem in the gut potentially lead to a rash, or even joint pain? Once again, it goes back to the concept of systems and symptoms.

The slightly contentious theory here regarding the gut causing systemic symptoms, is that having poor intestinal bacteria (or gut flora) leads to a phenomenon called increased intestinal permeability. This means that tight junctions (barrier defences in the lining of the gut wall) fail at doing their job of keeping the gut contents within the gut. If these tight junctions fail, they allow molecules from within the gut to filter out into the bloodstream through the gut wall.[35] This 'leak' of molecules into the bloodstream can then lead to inflammatory symptoms outside the gut, such as those mentioned above and more. This means SIBO is a gateway to various symptoms, but potentially also to 'autoimmunity'.[36] Autoimmunity is a phenomenon in which a person's immune system attacks their own organs and tissues. Examples include lupus, rheumatoid arthritis, psoriasis, multiple sclerosis, coeliac disease, thyroid disorders (Hashimoto's and Graves' diseases), myasthenia gravis, type 1 diabetes and polymyalgia rheumatica.

Autoimmunity can arise from:[37]

- a genetic predisposition

- an environmental trigger, such as stress, toxins or viruses

- increased intestinal permeability (theorised)

Both Amelia and Gary required a probiotic supplement for a while. This is because they both had a history of antibiotic use. I recommended the LGG® strain (*Lactobacillus GG* or *Lactobacillus rhamnosus*) because most of the studies on probiotics have focused on this one strain. It is naturally found in the gut, but becomes depleted by antibiotics. The balance of good and bad bacteria in the gut has an effect on our immune function and responses.

CHAPTER SUMMARY

- Several factors can affect the gastrointestinal tract beyond simply 'a healthy diet'.

- Someone's story will often give clues as to which areas may need addressing via their **Health Loop**.

- Small changes (removing one thing but adding in another) can provide huge gains.

- Increased intestinal permeability may lead to various symptoms and could potentially trigger autoimmunity.

- Remember: think **How, What and When?**

8

'I WANT TO BEAT THOSE ACHES AND PAINS'

One sign that we may have a new health issue to deal with is that we start to experience a symptom. Symptoms can vary, anything from pain to weight loss, discoloured nails or a racing heartbeat. Take pain, for example. You wake up one day with pain, and your immediate thought is to wonder why it's there. In the case of acute injury, like sprains and strains, it's obvious, and you can usually figure out if you've just 'slept funny' and given yourself a temporary pain in your neck. When it comes to longer-term pain, though, it's not as straightforward to identify and 'fix' the issue.

Pain is as fascinating as it is distressing. The way we experience it is totally individual and it is not always down to what we think it is.

This is borne out by many phenomena:

- patients who have normal MRI scans of their spine or other joints, but are in excruciating pain

- sportspersons who sustain a fracture during play but carry on regardless, often winning the match

- people who have dental extractions with no pain relief in certain parts of the world where they do not give pain any attention

The list goes on.

As you will have seen already, *The Health Fix* lays out a framework and gives you a toolkit that will help you feel better and can, in many cases, totally extinguish symptoms – and in my experience, this often goes for pain.

Take the case of Raphael. He is a thirty-two-year-old marketing manager with stiffness and joint pains. He aches most of the time and relies on massages from his partner, some NHS physiotherapy and ibuprofen tablets, which help a little. He has been told that he may have fibromyalgia by two doctors as well as a physiotherapist, as he is so debilitated at times.

When I first heard Raphael's symptoms, I was expecting a story of high stress, possibly a background of traumatic events and for lots of things to jump out at me from his **Health Loop**. This is often the case in patients with fibromyalgia or chronic pain.

But I could not have been more wrong.

Raphael had been feeling increasingly worse for the last four years. He'd had some blood tests under the care of another GP and his local hospital, which all came back perfectly normal, including the ones for rheumatic and autoimmune conditions. He also had normal X-rays. Aside from his pain, Raphael was happy and healthy. He actively managed any stress, had some great routines, like meditating, drinking lots of water, exercising regularly and eating a good, wholesome diet (way better than mine). He appeared to have had the most loving and nurturing upbringing one could imagine. He lived with his mum and dad, who had already told him about the importance of vitamin D,[38] particularly as they are of African-Caribbean origin.

Raphael's typical day consisted of getting up at 6am, drinking a pint of water and having a shower. He would then cycle to work and have breakfast, usually an oat-based bowl of cereal with a cup of tea. Interestingly, this would often make him feel tired, and his joints seemed to hurt for an hour or two afterwards.

He would then have a large salad for lunch, followed by an apple or two in the afternoon. Dinner was usually chicken or fish and vegetables; he followed a semi-low-carb-type diet in the evenings, as his mum had type 2 diabetes and was already on this regime (no potatoes, no bread, no pasta, no biscuits or sweets later in the day) to help control her blood sugar. About two hours before bed, he and his dad would usually have a sugar-free mug of cocoa.

Raphael went to the gym four times a week, mixing aerobic and weight-lifting workouts and his girlfriend had recently got him into mindfulness.

In terms of his medical history, there was really very little of note. He had always been as 'healthy as a horse' to use his own words, and his joints were normal, according to his medical examination.

I could tell that this was going to be a bit of a mystery, but I had *The Health Fix* toolkit in my head and I was going to stick to it.

As always, we started with the **Health Loop**.

Raphael's Health Loop

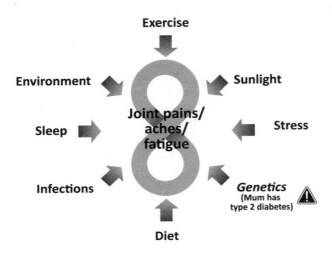

Drill Down and Diary Up

Now, what's interesting here is that there is nothing obvious in Raphael's **Health Loop**. When this happens, it's time to 'get out the drill'.

By this, I mean we need to drill down a bit more in certain areas to help us uncover what might be going on. I usually start by repeating the questions I've already asked about medical history and family illness in case I missed something. Once I'd done this with Raphael without uncovering anything new, I turned once more to his typical day and paid even closer attention to what he was telling me about his symptoms.

'Tell me more about your joint pains again, but give me a

flavour of when you get them – when they are at their worst and best?' I asked him.

He searched his brain for a few seconds. 'Er, OK... so... last weekend I was laid up in bed for a whole day with pain because it was so bad, and I hadn't even done anything. We'd been to my auntie's place and had a big family get together, then my girlfriend dropped me off home to my mum's, and a couple of hours later my ankles and my shoulders were killing me. Even ibuprofen didn't really help.'

'Hmm, interesting... what had you done that day? Any gym workout or, I dunno, hacking down trees or hedges in the garden? And what did you do at your aunt's?'

'Nothing. I did nothing in the morning, and went to hers for about twelve-thirty for lunch. She's an amazing cook. We had some of her goat curry, rice, peas, lentils... and then some creamy rum punch as a treat..'

'Hmm. Do you normally get joint pains after drinking alcohol?'

'No – not at all. I don't drink much, but when I do, alcohol doesn't ever flare up my joints.'

'OK. That's really useful. What about after having milk or cream?'

'Er... hmm... never really thought about that. Possibly. Actually, I do get pain after breakfast in the morning, and sometimes at night in bed – those are the only two times a day I have any milk, normally.'

So now that the drilling down may have paid off, it was time to bring out the diary.

The key is not to use the drill and the diary willy-nilly. So many people go off on wild goose chases. We had got to this point in Raphael's case because the **Health Loop** hadn't thrown up anything obvious, all of his tests for types of arthritis, gout and lupus were normal, and yet we still had an unresolved symptom.

'OK, can you keep a diary for me? I want you to keep a note of when you get your joint pains, and with that keep a record of what you are doing, where you are and what you eat and drink.

Then, after a week, I want you to cut out milk products from your diet, and we can touch base in a month if that's OK?'

ONE MONTH LATER

'Hi Raphael. How are you getting on?'

'Er. Yeah, good, I think... I didn't get any joint pains at all for two, maybe two and half weeks off the milk, but then out of the blue the other night, I got a huge flare-up again. I've been on my usual healthy diet, as you can see here from my notes, but I noticed that day I had a large salad with... hang on, hang on... I made a note... cucumber, chickpeas, tomatoes, kidney beans and onions. All in the salad. It couldn't be one of them causing it, could it? I mean... stopping the milk has really helped. I'm having mackerel, salmon or sardines on toast for breakfast now, with a cup of green or black tea.'

'Well it could be more than one thing. There are certain foods which contain high levels of a type of protein called lectins, including nightshade vegetables that might be responsible. They're healthy foods like peas, lentils, certain nuts and beans. But I don't really want you to stop eating them for no good reason.'

'Can I get tested for it? I don't mind paying.'

'Well, our NHS blood tests only show true allergies, and intolerance testing can be unreliable. Why don't you leave out some of the lectin-rich foods for a few weeks to see if it helps, then we can touch base again. I will send you a list of foods that you can have and the ones to avoid so you can plan meals. Then, after that, we can reintroduce them, one by one, to see what happens.'

A month later, Raphael's joint pains had all but gone. It was remarkable. He had got his life back.

There are a few points to take note of in Raphael's case. Firstly, I do not advocate messing around with diets unless there is good reason to. In this case, we only explored it as part of the **Drill Down and Diary Up** exercise after his **Health Loop** drew a blank. (I hasten to add that this exercise may not always reveal something. There are conditions such as Lyme disease, lupus, connective tissue disorders and syphilis that often mimic other conditions and can be hard to diagnose.)

Secondly, Raphael was really activated. Like Amelia and Gary (and unlike some of the people you will meet later in the book), he didn't need any motivating. No **IDEAL** framework required. Many people would struggle with a change in diet, but he found it remarkably easy.

Thirdly, not everyone needs to stop drinking cow's milk and start avoiding lectins! I am not in the business of villainizing whole foods. Interestingly, the healthier your microbiome, the more likely you are to be able to tolerate a variety of foods – and it's self-fulfilling, because a broad variety of foods helps maintain a healthy microbiome.

Finally, Raphael had been seen by several GPs and a specialist, meaning he had explored a whole barrage of different tests, all of which returned normal results, before we went down this route.

Deep dive: Allergy and inflammation

There are two phenomena going on here with Raphael. The first is his 'reaction' to milk. Broadly speaking, there are two types of allergy to milk – IgE and non-IgE. The first is when the immune system makes an antibody called IgE, which latches on to the casein protein in milk and causes a variety of symptoms, like rashes, sickness, a blocked nose and breathing difficulties. In severe cases, it can lead to a potentially life-threatening allergic reaction called anaphylaxis.

Non-IgE mediated allergy is milder, with no antibody being involved, but instead a partial response from the immune system. In this case, the symptoms take longer to manifest and are less severe. In Raphael's case, I am not actually sure if it was non-IgE allergy at play (joint pains are not a classic symptom), or whether he was simply triggering inflammation via another mechanism each time he consumed milk, either in his tea, his cereal, or in his aunt's milk-based punch.[39] It begs the question: how did this issue arise in the first place?

In Raphael's case, he'd had joint pains on and off for four years, but as yet, there was no detectable damage to his joints. He was generally healthy, so it is likely that his reaction to milk happened because he was eliciting a partial immune response in his joints each time he consumed it.

How does this happen? It's hard to say for sure, but one theory is called molecular mimicry.[40] This is a case of mistaken identity, where the immune system identifies part of a protein (in this case, the casein in milk), sees it as a threat, and activates a partial immune response. For Raphael, this manifested as pain in his joints each time he consumed it.

In simple terms, it's like a police officer looking to arrest a criminal with a particular description – six feet tall, stocky build, fair skin, blond hair, wears a flat cap – but he ends up cuffing the wrong person: someone who matches *almost* all of that description, but is actually totally innocent. Remove the 'innocent' milk, in this case, and the problem of mistaken identity disappears. A good example of this is birch pollen and oral allergy syndrome which overlap. If you get a swollen lip whenever you eat certain fruits, such as uncooked cherries and apples, you are probably also allergic to birch pollen, as the protein molecules in certain fruits look similar to those in birch pollen.[41]

The second issue for Raphael was possibly lectins. This is controversial, as lectin foods are nutritious and have many benefits, but they are also seen by some as anti-nutrients. Potatoes, lentils, kidney beans, tomatoes, peas, peanuts and aubergines are all lectins. Most people have no issue with them, but in susceptible individuals, they can cause joint pain and digestive discomfort, such as bloating. The jury is out as to whether lectins actually play a part in the development of autoimmune conditions, but in Raphael's case, eliminating some of them seemed to help.[42]

It's also worth noting that a key part of muscle and joint health is movement and exercise, but you can read more about this in the Fixes section. Raphael was already exercising regularly, so there were no concerns in that area.

CHAPTER SUMMARY

- If nothing obvious shows up in your **Health Loop** remember to **Drill Down and Diary Up** as you revisit each area – diet, exercise, environment, genetics, sunlight, infections, stress and sleep.

- A simple way to work out if you are reacting to a particular food is simply by being aware of how you feel an hour or two after you have eaten. Keep a diary. Look out for bloating, pain, brain fog or fatigue.

- If you identify a food that makes you feel unwell, then it may be worth trying an elimination diet for a month to see if you feel better.

8

'I WANT TO IMPROVE MY MOOD, AND FEEL CALM AND FOCUSED'

This is arguably one of the hardest of challenges in the world in which we live today. I mentioned earlier that not a day in my clinical practice goes by without someone presenting with a gut issue, but the same goes for people making contact about their mental or emotional health. If you have never experienced depression,[43] anxiety,[44] grief or emotional turmoil for a prolonged period of time, then you must count yourself lucky.

This is taken verbatim from the World Health Organization website:

Mental health conditions are increasing worldwide. Mainly because of demographic changes, there has been a 13% rise in mental health conditions and substance use disorders in the last decade (to 2017). Mental health conditions now cause 1 in 5 years lived with disability. Around 20% of the world's children and adolescents have a mental health condition, with suicide the second leading cause of death among 15–29-year-olds.[45]

Mental health is such a broad term.[46] In some ways, I guess it means anything that is not considered to be physical health. But if we think about the concept of systems and symptoms once more, all of our systems are involved in our *health*, whether that be physical or mental.

There are many ways to think about mental health, just as there are many ways to explain what depression and anxiety are, or where they come from.

Here's an odd exercise. Imagine you actually wanted to make someone feel anxious. What would you do? Take away their home? Hurl a load of abuse at them, perhaps? You might fuel their stress by stealing from them, or you might deny them food and drink – or do the opposite and allow them only junk food, get them to drink too much alcohol and coffee, and then maybe deprive them of sleep. This slightly vulgar exercise reveals just a handful of things that can drive our mental health symptoms – and this can help us understand the inputs that affect us.

Sometimes it can be helpful to use metaphors to illustrate certain concepts, as this can help people better understand and manage their condition. For instance, take the familiar explanation about our fight-or-flight response (i.e. this is what happens to us when a tiger jumps out at us from behind a tree). This is a useful one to explain what happens during a panic attack or moments of extreme anxiety. Your heart rate goes up, your mouth runs dry and your adrenaline shoots through the roof, getting you ready to run for your life – which is exactly what you would need to be doing if a tiger jumped out at you.

Replace that tiger with a bad boss or a constant stream of stressful emails, and you might be experiencing this reaction several times a day: that's anxiety. It's the same fear response caused by the tiger behind the tree, but this response is totally inappropriate if it kicks off when you're at home or in a work meeting (as opposed to, say, the Sundarbans National Park in West Bengal, where a tiger really might jump out at you).

It's good to remember that the tools we can use to help ourselves are often things we do each day. As you will have seen by now, small changes can make big differences.

In a moment, I am going to tell you about Shane, who was at the brink with his mental health. Everyone's story is unique, but his is particularly interesting; there are so many facets to how he got to this point in his life, and to what allowed him to move forward. If we accept one of my two definitions of 'lifestyle' – that it is a combination of luck and habits – Shane certainly had his share of bad luck.

'I don't even know why I'm here, really. I just didn't know where else to go...' Shane paused and gently crumpled into tears. I had glanced at his notes on screen before he came into the room, and could see that he was eighteen years old.

'It's OK, it's all right. Take your time,' I said.

'Basically... well... basically, I pretty much tried to kill myself last night. My life is just... well... awful. I'm sleeping in the back of a van that isn't even mine, I haven't had a shower in two weeks, I've got no money... I'm... like... properly finished.'

Shane had left school at sixteen and started working at a builders' yard. He'd been fired about six months ago with no warning, and had starting doing a bit of work for his older brother, but that had dried up. He was now sleeping in his brother's old van, as his brother's partner had just had a baby (they were living in a one-bed flat across town). Shane's mum and stepdad lived not too far away, but they had fallen out with both him and his brother, after what sounded like quite a torrid and abusive relationship. The brothers had both been told never to come back to the house.

Shane had tried to take his own life by half-heartedly cutting his wrists in the back of the van, but he had just not been able to bring himself to 'do it properly'. He regretted it, but felt totally stuck. His friends were all working or at college, and he had lost touch with them.

It was heartbreaking listening to Shane's story. He was comfort eating, living off chocolate bars he'd loved as a school kid and processed snacks, mainly from petrol stations, where he would go to use the toilets. He had stayed on his brother's sofa for a couple of nights, but the lack of space meant he felt he had overstayed his welcome.

In situations like these, a person's needs around safety and basic provisions[47] are so immediate that those all need sorting out before any further exploration of background symptoms can be carried out. After a forty-five-minute consultation and several phone calls, Shane was safe, knowing he had a bed for the night, and I arranged to see him again in a few days, as he was clearly at risk of harm.

When he came back, he was looking better but still feeling very low. He confessed that he had been feeling low and anxious for some time, ever since he'd left school. He had lost touch with his two best friends, and his home situation was unstable, with a lot of disruption from a young age. His mum had been quite depressed when he was young, and had been in and out of hospital with it. His stepdad was alcohol-dependent and aggressive. Shane had also been bullied at school for years.

In fact, he had a full house of factors to set the scene for poor health and wellbeing. Almost all of these were totally out of his control. These factors are often referred to as ACEs – or adverse childhood experiences – and they can have a huge impact on one's health.[48]

At a glance, Shane's **Health Loop** looks similar to many others, but the approach here was to start with the most important issues, like making sure he actually had food to eat and a roof over his head. Once we'd addressed these issues, we could start to deal with his background needs, which would enable him to feel better.

Shane's Health Loop

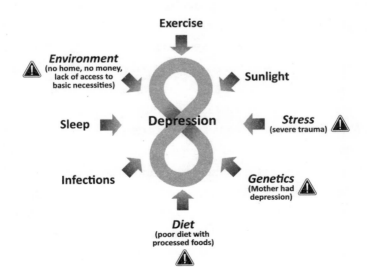

Shane had been on antidepressant medication briefly as a teenager, at the suggestion of a child psychiatrist. It helped him initially, but he had stopped it after he started to get headaches and felt tired. He was very keen not to take any medication this time. He'd also found the process of counselling really difficult when he had attended sessions in years gone by, and initially declined it when I brought it up.

I sent Shane for some blood tests to check his physical health, as that can sometimes unwittingly be ignored when mental health is the main issue. Thankfully, his results all came back as optimal.

In the back of my mind, once we had got some of the basics in place, I felt that Shane could really benefit from some health coaching. For those who know what health coaches do, they have, in my opinion, been the missing piece in the NHS[49] for many years. They are experts in understanding what matters to a person and tailoring behaviour-change suggestions to help people look after themselves.

Most NHS GP surgeries now have access to a health coach, but when Shane came to see me, we did not have such access, nor did we have access to social prescribers, who can help signpost if someone has health issues underpinned by a social problem.

What there was access to at the time was social services, Citizen's Advice and free group counselling sessions via a local voluntary organisation, which he eventually agreed to attend.

The marvellous thing about Shane was that he was very open to changing his habits. He just hadn't had the opportunity before now to even try. He had been in an unfortunate situation, which meant he had become totally deconditioned. If you go without experiencing something for long enough, whether that be love, compassion or fresh food, you almost forget what it's like. Once Shane had his basics – food, warmth, hot water and the like – he needed gentle support, plus a community who could help him rebuild his confidence and restore his purpose, which was to become a builder.

I caught up with Shane every few weeks, and the changes in him were remarkable (we'll cover them shortly).

One of the areas he and I had talked about was a word that grates on me a little – resilience – and how to build it.

'Vulnerable but invincible'

The word resilience in modern times comes from the 1970s research work of Dr Emmy Werner[50] involving a group of children from the Hawaiian island of Kauai. She actually uses the word 'resiliency'. The group of children she studied all had ACEs like Shane – troubled childhoods with significant amounts of trauma. Dr Werner's findings showed that the children who went on to become happy adults had certain factors in common (including good emotional support, autonomy, sociability and willingness to take opportunities). And I personally love the phrase Dr Werner used to describe the children in her study who were found to be resilient: 'vulnerable but invincible'.

The reason that ACEs are so important is that a failure to acknowledge them can mean the person affected may go on to have difficulty coping with their emotions and end up causing themselves or others harm – and that ties directly into their behaviours.

For instance, adults who as children did not get meals or had erratic mealtimes may have quite a different relationship with food to those who had very regimented mealtimes. In the same way, a child who did not receive much affection in their early years may find attachments more difficult, or come across to others as emotionally cold as an adult.

In any case, when we think about Shane, he had suffered a lot of childhood trauma. Thinking about the factors that lead to resilience, he had now managed to find some good emotional support via his group. He had made friends, and they had begun to support each other.

Not only that, but Shane had a lot of opportunities come his way through this new network, including help getting his CV together for the first time and applying for work at a big chain of retail stores. He also ended up living with a member of the group in shared accommodation, and that is when he learned how to cook. After a couple of months, he was even laughing and cracking jokes when he came back to see me.

His transformation really was quite something to witness – a total metamorphosis, predominantly because he had managed to change his environment.

Environment was the biggest issue in Shane's life (and hence in his **Health Loop**). And, as we have seen with the **Drawstring Effect**, once his environment changed and he got some support, his stress levels came down and his mood dramatically improved. Shane was already quite a fit person, and actually the other parts of his **Health Loop** did not need much attention.

Let's just think about Shane's changes briefly.

Symptom	Changes	Benefits
Bad environment	Finding a new home, becoming part of a community and making friends	Lower stress, better sleep, a space to learn to cook, improved concentration, the ability to find work
Poor diet	Learning to cook	Improve mood, gut health, energy and self-esteem

You will see here that each part of this grid basically tightened things up further. The cooking, for instance, was a result of his flatmate's influence, but it then improved Shane's diet, which led to improvement in his mood, and he felt less stressed.

If we think about what is happening in the background here, it's all rather powerful. Even if we look at just one aspect of health, such as immunity, we know from research that our thoughts, food, sleep and companionship can all support it.

In terms of Shane's **Lifestyle Prescription**, there were still some practices that he held on to that had helped him from when he was homeless, such as not wasting anything or leaving any drink or meal unfinished, but in his case, no **How, What and When** adjustments were necessary.

For focus and 'being in the moment' to get him away from negative thoughts, I asked Shane to try my one-minute recharge once a day (see page 67), and I also gave him this exercise for adding positive flips to negative thoughts.

Flip exercise

This exercise seems a little inane, but it forces someone to generate a response to a negative thought. I often start people off on this before going down the road of more conventional cognitive behavioural therapy (CBT – see below). It just gets the brain used to searching for an alternative to the negative thought, however ridiculous it may seem.

For example, for the negative thought, 'I've got nothing going for me,' the positive flip might be, 'Actually, I'm still pretty good at football – maybe I'll play again one day.' This is not to be confused with toxic positivity. It's simply a way of making your brain generate another possible outcome. Not everyone is a fan, but it can help get people out of a repetitive cycle of 'stinking thinking' quite quickly.

Think different, feel different – but how?

The way CBT[51] works is that each time you think a negative thought or use negative self-talk, e.g. 'You're useless' or 'You've let everyone down', you challenge that question or idea, realise that it is based on false beliefs about yourself (often stuck on you by family or friends) and then challenge it. As I've explained, our habits become us if we are not careful, and we can become labelled – or label ourselves. But our negative thoughts are often based on what are known as cognitive distortions. Here are some common distortions and examples of how they might be expressed. Most of these distortions related strongly to Shane when I first met him.

- **Overgeneralisation**: 'I am *always* bad at exams.'

- **All-or-nothing thinking**: 'I am a terrible musician.'

- **Discounting the positives**: 'I just about got through that interview – I guess they'll take anyone these days.'

- **Minimising or maximising**: 'Julian easily scored the best goal. Everyone must have seen me miss my shot.'

- **Emotional reasoning**: 'I felt ashamed, so I must have been coming across badly.'

- **Personalising**: 'No one enjoyed the party because I organised it.'

- **Labelling**: 'I lost my jacket. I'm a fool.'

- **Being hard on yourself**: 'I should have worked even harder.'

- **Conclusion shopping**: 'She said she couldn't make dinner last night. She must hate me.'

- **Filtering out the good**: 'I achieved nothing this week.'

Being aware of these is the first challenge, as all are quite monkey-brain driven, but if you step back and take an extra second, you can notice when you have thoughts like these. How many of the examples above ring true to you? All of them? A few of them? Maybe none.

The second challenge is about unpacking these distortions and reframing them.

A quick way is to do this:

- Say 'STOP' to yourself (visualise a big 'stop' sign if that helps).

- Ask yourself:
  - Am I looking at this in a black and white way? (Yes, most likely.)
  - What evidence do I have that this is even true? (None or not a lot, usually.)

- Generate an alternative thought, e.g. 'I lost my jacket – it'll probably turn up. Things like this happen now and again. Let me go and look for it...'

This is a very quick type of CBT; it's a bit of a shortcut and doesn't use journalling (which is by far my preferred way to do it, if one can invest the time).

The only part of Shane's **Health Loop** we have not covered is his family history. None of us can change our genes, but we can change how they are expressed. The simple, if slightly clichéd, explanation of genes loading your gun but your environment pulling the trigger springs to mind again. In other words, you may have propensity to a particular illness, yet never suffer from it, depending on many things, including your environment, luck and your habits.

The 'Genetics' thread of the **Health Loop** can be telling. In Shane's case, his mother had been hospitalised for severe depression. This is a rarer occurrence these days than in the 1980s and 90s,[52] thanks to crisis and outreach teams, but it is nevertheless a significant part of Shane's story.

Deep Dive: 'It runs in the family...'

Our genes tell a story. There are many genes – or rather parts of our genes called polymorphisms – that code for a predisposition to many conditions, including depression,[53] which we are focusing on here, but also things like coeliac disease, heart disease, vitamin D deficiency, ADHD or Alzheimer's disease.

Remember that genetics is only one of the strands of the **Health Loop**. If you do have a relevant family history, it should not be seen as a fait accompli that you will also have the condition, but nor should it be ignored.

If we look at depression – what it is and what causes it – we are often told that it is a constant feeling of sadness that can be caused by:

- brain chemistry disruption

- hormonal imbalance

- substances (drugs and alcohol)

- medical conditions and pain

- brain structural issues

- family history

- childhood trauma

You will notice some items on this list featured in Shane's story, including a family history of depression. There is no doubt that medication can be helpful for several of the causes of depression in that list, but the bottom line is this: whether it's an unlucky imbalance of your serotonin, dopamine, GABA and glutamate levels (i.e. brain chemistry), or the fact that you take cocaine and get terrible come-downs afterwards, or that you are in the throes of menopause, or that you have a long-term physical health condition, you are likely to benefit from building your own *Health Fix* toolkit.

For instance, I have seen several cases of depression that were improved just by someone prioritising sleep, or starting gentle exercise, or taking vitamin D (things that stood out as needing attention in those people's **Health Loops**). The point is – and I am sure of this by now – what you have read so far will convince you that it's never just one thing that leads to our illness or wellbeing, which is exactly why we need to lay out our story and look at everything with a bird's-eye view, but also an eagle eye when necessary.

Genetic testing is not currently a standard part of medical care, but is likely to become so in future. It needs a lot of thinking through in terms of ethics and requires counselling before testing. I remember seeing the 1997 film *Gattaca* as a medical student; the story is based in a fictional world of selection via genetic superiority, and the film blew my mind in terms of the ethical dilemmas it raised. DNA analysis or genetic testing can give us a range of information, some of which is of limited use, and some of which is critical.

An example of information of more limited use might be that someone, myself being one of them, is missing a gene such as MCM6, which aids the digestion of lactose,[54] but a critical one would be the BRCA1 or BRCA2 genes for someone with a family history of breast cancer.[55] The flip side is that many people may not want to know if they are going to develop certain conditions. For instance, James Watson, one of the scientists who discovered DNA, sequenced his own DNA but did not want to know whether he had an increased risk of developing Alzheimer's disease.[56]

As a side note, one group of NHS patients I have found who occasionally come in and ask about gene testing are women who have suffered the trauma of recurrent miscarriage. They occasionally ask for testing for a gene variation called MTHFR, which is the name of one of the genes as well as an enzyme responsible for methylation,[57] a cellular process involved in the regulation of folic acid levels as well as the breakdown of an amino acid in the blood called homocysteine. High levels of homocysteine can contribute to the development of both heart disease and Alzheimer's disease. While there is no direct cause and effect, women with a defective version of the MTHFR gene are more likely to experience miscarriage. More thought needs to be given around the future role of knowing more about our genes and the impact they may have on our health.

The most important thing to remember is that our genes are not necessarily our destiny. As I've explained, how our genes get expressed (as in whether they exert an effect on our health) is linked to our habits and our environment.

As for Shane, the changes he made and tools he learnt meant that he was ultimately able to thrive. He went on to become a supplies manager for a builders' merchant. He still has his ups and downs, but is far better able to manage them.

CHAPTER SUMMARY

- Mental health is complex, and there is usually no one cause or immediate fix for conditions like depression and anxiety.

- Negative feelings often come from negative thoughts, which are often known as cognitive distortions.

- The brain is capable of changing its function through behavioural techniques like CBT, and making other changes that can be clearly highlighted by examining your **Health Loop**.

- Our genetics play a part in many medical conditions, including mental health.

- One-minute recharges and breathing practices (particularly slow belly breathing, see page 178) can be helpful, as this stimulates your vagus nerve, making you feel relaxed and allowing you to be in the moment.

8

'I WANT TO DEAL WITH THESE MYSTERY SYMPTOMS'

At the beginning of this book, I mentioned that *The Health Fix* is really about the long game and is not aimed at acute medical problems. Acute medicine is when someone needs rapid assessment and treatment. Conditions like pneumonia, infections, ulcers, heart attack, stroke, asthma attacks, sepsis, suicidal intent and anaphylaxis (life-threatening allergic reaction) are urgent and need treating quickly. In an ideal world, we would be able to prevent these from happening, but that is not always possible.

But what about someone who is generally healthy and doing all that they can, but still keeps falling ill?

Could it be that there is something they are getting too much of that is making them unwell (e.g. cigarette smoke, certain foods, the wrong type of exercise or an unhealthy environment)? Or could it be that they are lacking something (e.g. micronutrients, oestrogen, emotional fulfilment or purpose)?

TOO MUCH of X? + TOO LITTLE of Y? = illness?

There are many examples of this, but I want to share Norah's story. She had been unwell for a year, and her experience illustrates two things. Firstly, that the **Health Loop** is generic. It can be used on anyone yet what it generates is something quite specific for each person. Secondly, that the answer is almost always rooted in the patient's story.

Norah was twenty-nine and working as a trainee accountant. She had moved down to the south of England from her family home in Scotland a year before, and had not felt well since. She was 'a total health freak' (her words) and, as well as being an ex-county level runner, was a paragon of wellbeing.

Her symptoms were varied and included headaches, brain fog, dizziness, an occasional fast heart rate, electric-shock-type feelings down her arms, nausea and one episode of fainting. She had seen a number of doctors privately through her work's health insurance, and they had all told her everything was within normal limits. When I met her, she had already had full blood works done, including full blood count, tests for kidney and liver function, coeliac screening, and tests for vitamins D and B12. She'd had iron studies and copper studies (caeruloplasmin). They'd tested her magnesium, and also carried out an autoimmune screen, ESR and a CRP. She had also had an MRI scan of her brain, an ECG trace and echo test of her heart (to look at its pumping function), and an endoscopy (a camera test to look down her stomach). All of these had come back normal.

Norah was at a total loss, and, to be honest, I was worried I may not be able to help her, as she had clearly already been investigated thoroughly.

When I looked at her results, I noticed that her CRP, a blood marker for inflammation or infection, was slightly raised (fifteen). This is still deemed normal, but can be a marker of inflammation (or, if very high, infection). I will come back to this, as it could be an important clue as to what might be going on.

And so we embarked on Norah's *Health Fix* journey. What was fascinating about Norah is that she had effectively already been through it all herself, and had already made some big changes in her life.

'That's why I'm so annoyed about this,' she told me. 'About three years ago, I was overweight and had come out of a bad relationship. I thought I'd get my life back on track. I knew I had to change something, so I started doing our local Parkrun, joined a book group, changed my diet, and changed my job – and I'd been feeling fine ever since, until about a year ago. I just don't get it. What am I doing wrong, doc? Do you think it's something serious like cancer, but somehow all the tests are just coming back normal?'

Norah had already effectively done the **IDEAL** framework on herself by making changes to her lifestyle, and for a while she had felt the power of the **Drawstring Effect**, but now here she was, suddenly feeling quite unwell again, and nothing was working.

Her **Health Loop** looked pretty unremarkable.

Norah's Health Loop

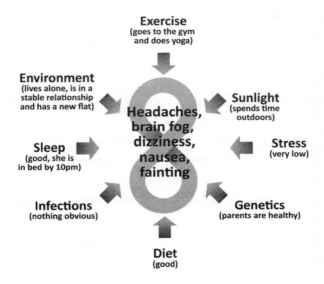

This, of course, meant it was time to **Drill Down and Diary Up**.

'OK. We need to really drill down on your symptoms. You say that all the specialists have reassured you, right?'

'Yeah. Which I'm pleased about, but I still feel rough. I know something's not right.'

'I know, I can imagine it's frustrating. Could you keep a diary of your symptoms? We need to be able to see exactly when they come on, how long they last, and so on. And also if you notice anything related to things like sleep, mealtimes, that sort of thing.'

Four weeks later, we touched base after Norah had emailed me her diary.

10–17 July

Monday – Woke up, muzzy head, heart racing, work, felt fine until home. Felt ill after 7pm.

Tuesday – Woke up feeling sick, headache. Fine at work. Ate fruit only. Went for short run until 7pm. Felt awful again after 8pm.

Wednesday – Woke up with muzzy head, extremely tired. Not too bad at work. Home by 6pm. Felt ill after 7pm.

Thursday – Missed early 7am meeting, feeling electric-shock pain and nausea. Again eased off during day. Worse again in the evening.

Friday – Took day off work with exhaustion. Felt unwell all day in bed.

Saturday – Went to brother's house near Bristol. Felt quite well, stayed overnight.

Sunday – At brother's house. Felt well until I went back home and went to bed.

At this point, it was obvious to both of us that she felt ill for certain parts of the day, but that it seemed to ease off when she was at work. And she didn't feel ill at her brother's house.

'Do you think it's something in my house that's making me ill?' she said. 'I read something in the *Daily Mail* about this woman who had illness caused by mould, but she had rashes as well. Could it be something like that?'

'Well, I'm not sure, to be honest. But given your diary, it is pretty likely to be something in your home environment. Have you got a gas boiler, by any chance?'

'Er, yeah. Why?'

'I just wonder whether you may have carbon monoxide poisoning.'

The rest is history.

In a way, this all seems obvious, but it had crept up on Norah indolently and, as in so many other cases, her symptoms were down to her environment. If we go back to the formula we looked at at the start of the chapter (too much of X + too little of Y = illness), we can see that the 'too much' in this case was a toxin, namely carbon monoxide. There was nothing clever here beyond good diary keeping. Within a week of getting her boiler fixed, Norah's health had started to improve and she was back on track. She hadn't spotted that she was only ill at home because of her outdoorsy lifestyle, coupled with the fact that she was often out of the house and also lived alone.

A story of too much

I remember a frustrated copywriter who had long-term prostatitis (inflammation of the prostate) with only little relief of his symptoms after both medical massage by a urologist and several long courses of antibiotics like Ciprofloxacin. His **Health Loop** revealed that he ate six – yes six – blocks of cheese daily. You can guess the rest of the story. His symptoms improved dramatically after ditching the cheese, purely based on the 'too much' theory and nothing else.

You'll remember that one interesting thing I'd noticed in Norah's blood tests was her levels of CRP (or C-reactive protein). This can be a marker of inflammation or infection, and to me it suggested that she was inflamed.

Deep Dive: How does inflammation actually arise? The triad.

Long-term or chronic inflammation is different to the acute (sudden and short-lived) inflammation most of us get from time to time when suffering from things like sprained ankles, insect bites or a viral sore throat.

Chronic inflammation is a result of a process called oxidative stress,[58] where our bodies produce free radicals (also known as reactive oxygen species). They occur when an oxygen molecule (O_2) splits into two single atoms. These atoms are unstable and are produced as part of the ageing process, but also in response to how we live (things like smoking, poor diet, high stress, exposure to toxins, too much exercise, etc.). Unlike stable molecules, which have pairs of electrons, these free radicals are now missing an electron.

This means they seek to react with other compounds by stealing one of their electrons, thereby turning these other cells into free radicals themselves. This starts a chain reaction of sorts, with more free-radical production, which damages our cells and our DNA, eventually leading to our immune system being unable to cope with the free radicals if left unchecked.

This diagram shows the triad that occurs in the development of long-term disease.

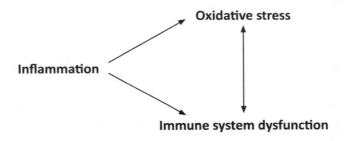

This process of damage or oxidation (I sometimes think of it like the rust on metal or the browning of a bitten apple) is linked to long-term or chronic inflammation, and also to many diseases, such as heart disease, Alzheimer's disease and cancer.[59]

One way of trying to combat free-radical damage is to ensure a high intake of what are known as antioxidant-rich foods, which provide electrons to these free radicals, effectively mopping them up and thereby preventing damage to our cells. These foods include fruits and vegetables like carrots, sweet potatoes, berries, spinach and peppers, as well as green tea, coffee and dark chocolate.[60]

Unsurprisingly, other methods include managing stress, regular movement and exercise, and prioritising sleep. There is a key link here between what is happening at a cellular level and the concept of symptoms and system malfunction.

Commonality in disease processes

Biologically, this triad of inflammation, oxidative stress and immune dysfunction features in almost all non-communicable diseases (diseases we don't catch from other people) such as those mentioned on the previous page. The processes in the triad slowly snowball as we move from symptoms towards developing an established disease. But notice in the diagram below that all the flow arrows in the diagram are two-way. And this means that many symptoms are amenable to change until the point where the triad processes become overwhelming and cannot easily, if at all, be 'reversed'.

When our hospital specialist colleagues come to chat to our GP teams to share the latest in their various worlds of expertise, they will often flash up slides on mechanisms of anything from the latest drug therapy in osteoporosis, to the prevention of recurrent early miscarriage, or even potential Alzheimer's disease treatments.

What is striking is how often near identical some of their respective slides are in terms of the mechanisms that they display – they all feature this triad in various guises whether it be proteins like NFkappaB or arachidonic acid pathways for inflammation.

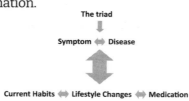

In Norah's case, the inflammation had an external source – carbon monoxide poisoning – and the source simply needed to be removed in order for her to regain her health. As we know and have seen, inflammogens (i.e. things that cause inflammation) in everyday life include air pollution, stress, highly processed foods, smoking and excess alcohol.

CHAPTER SUMMARY

- The timing of symptoms may be of importance, and a diary can be useful to help you spot patterns here.

- Think about the principle of 'too much' vs 'too little'. Is there something you can remove that may be hindering your health, or something you can add in to support it? If you do both, the effect is magnified.

- Long-term inflammation is damaging to us and needs addressing. Think of easy ways to incorporate simple changes into your routine that may help, as inflammation tends to increase with time and age if left unchecked.

8

'I WANT A SHARPER MEMORY'

Hardly a week goes by in my work when I don't come across someone who is struggling with concentration or memory. As I mentioned before, these chapter titles are based on some of the most common 'health wishes' I hear. At the deep end of faltering memory is dementia, which is a syndrome primarily affecting the brain that eventually affects a person's ability to function in many other ways. It often manifests with memory problems.

The statistics make grim reading: 'Globally, the numbers of people living with dementia will increase from 50m in 2018 to 152m in 2050, a 204% increase.'[61]

Dementia is a specific term, and most cases are down to Alzheimer's disease or vascular dementia. In Alzheimer's disease, there is a build-up of tangles in the brain called 'tau tangles', the formation of which is triggered by a protein called amyloid. The disease can run in families. Vascular dementia ('vascular' meaning relating to blood vessels) is similar to heart disease in that it results from the blood supply to the brain being compromised by diseased arteries that become clogged up, thereby effectively starving the brain of oxygen and nutrients. A stroke is an example of the kind of event that may lead to vascular dementia.

But not all memory issues immediately imply dementia. I know friends and patients in their thirties, forties and fifties who have brain fog and memory issues frequently. The good news is that, in many cases, there is a lot that can be done to improve this.

Janine's story illustrates this well.

Janine was forty-four. She had three young children, no current partner, and worked as a secretary in a private hospital. She found herself forgetting names and faces as well as important tasks at work.

By now, you will probably have got the sense that, out of all of our systems, I think the brain is arguably the most important. Just to recap, the reason for this is that even if you crack the code of your **Health Loop**, you still have to activate yourself to make the changes, for instance by using my **IDEAL** framework (see page 26). But even this means changing your habits, which means changing how you think, which means you hand over the keys to your brain. But what if you feel like your brain is not working properly? This is what Janine was experiencing.

'Tell me about your typical day.'

'Well, I'm up early – around six-thirty – but I'm already exhausted. I get the kids up and out of bed, we all grab breakfast, usually toast and cereal, and we're ready to leave the house by eight. Once I've dropped them off, I get to work around nine. They're really good with my hours, so sometimes I get in for nine-thirty. Roni, my youngest, had leukaemia a few years ago, so I'm always on tenterhooks in case the school rings to say he has a fever or something. I tend to get food from the canteen at work. It's a pretty good selection. I always get a proper meal – we get a massive staff discount. I can get a pie, chips and peas, or a ploughman's with crisps, for three quid. For the last few months, I've been really struggling – literally falling asleep at my desk and not able to remember anything. My brain just isn't *working*. It really scares me, especially as my dad had Alzheimer's. One day, I forgot to send some important outpatient letters, which I usually do every week at the same time. I really hate this feeling, because I like doing a good job. I drink a lot of sweet, milky coffee to keep me going. Teas and coffees are free at work, so that's useful.

'My mum picks up the kids from school a few times a week, and on those days, I get home and have a nap. Otherwise, it's straight to school pick-up or after-school club, and then home. We normally have tea at around six. The kids are good eaters, so I'm lucky I guess. I usually treat myself with some crisps or a chocolate bar later on in front of the telly. We normally have something easy I can slam in the oven, like a fish pie or chicken goujons with some mixed vegetables. My eldest, Dania, is really helpful and helps me sort out Rafi and Roni for bed. Then I usually help Dania with her homework – she's in year eight now – but I can't focus recently. I feel bad. I thought it might be alcohol making me groggy, but I haven't had a drink in about two months now. I'm often exhausted, and I have to say I tend to feel a bit low. I'd never do anything silly, but I just feel a bit shut down. No real reason. I've got no stress or other big worries at the moment. Money's been a bit tight recently, but we manage all right. It's almost like my brain has just switched off. Luckily, I work for a neurology consultant, and I told her about it all, so she quickly arranged a brain scan. That came back totally normal, so I know I don't have a tumour or a stroke or anything like that. But she said I should definitely see you.'

Janine was an excellent storyteller, and as I listened, I had been busy mentally filling in her **Health Loop**.

Janine's Health Loop

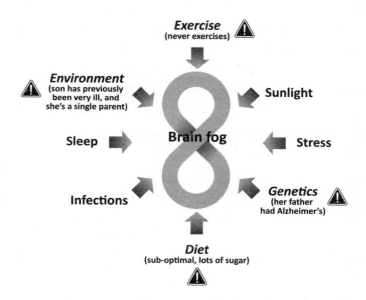

Janine's story was interesting. There was so much in there – and, as with most people, a lot of shades of grey. She was quite content, really, but felt her brain was suddenly letting her down. The other overriding theme in her story was that she was constantly on high alert, always thinking about her children with little time for herself.

Physically, Janine felt she was overweight (she had put on 5kg in the past year) but otherwise, I was struck by how young she looked for her age. I arranged for some blood tests, which revealed that she had a borderline low B12 level, and also that she was peri-menopausal and had pre-diabetes. This, in some ways, was quite satisfying, as it gave us something to work with beyond what was in her **Health Loop**.

Before we move on to Janine's **Lifestyle Prescription**, it might be useful to revisit the systems at play:

- gastrointestinal system

- immune system

- endocrine (hormones) and reproductive system

- nervous system (brain)

- cardiovascular system

- musculoskeletal system

All these systems are interconnected, so although Janine's main symptoms are brain-based, the changes she needs to make will involve the other systems rather than just focusing on the brain itself. We know, for instance, that she is low on B12, and we also know her blood glucose levels are running high, as she is bordering on type 2 diabetes, while her oestrogen levels are waning. All of these factors are implicated in brain function.[62][63][64]

In fact, a standard dementia screen should always include blood tests for B12 levels and diabetes.

Deep dive: Alzheimer's disease

Alzheimer's disease is not a pleasant prospect. I have seen the effect it has on families and carers at close quarters. While it is unlikely that the condition can be made totally preventable, there is no doubt there are many triggers that, if we box clever, we can do our best to avoid. My philosophy is that if I am going to develop a condition like Alzheimer's, I would much rather it appear at the age of eighty than at sixty.

In Janine's case, her father had Alzheimer's, and this was very much one of her concerns when it came to her memory. Alzheimer's disease is on the rise.[65] As explained earlier, Alzheimer's disease involves the formation of 'tau tangles' in the brain. The clues as to why this happens to an individual can be found in their **Health Loop** which includes genetics.

We inherit twenty-three chromosomes from each of our biological parents. Chromosomes are made up of genes, which are made up of DNA. Within these genes are variations called alleles. Each person inherits at least one allele from each parent for each of their genes.

How genetic inheritance of alleles works

Mum

	a	a
A	Aa	Aa
a	aa	aa

Dad

In the case of Alzheimer's, the gene that seems to play the biggest role in leading to the disease is called APOE. This gene is responsible for providing instructions for making a protein called apolipoprotein E, which carries fats through the bloodstream. There are three versions of this gene (or alleles): APOE2, APOE3 and APOE4. The APOE3 variant is the commonest type, found in 50% of people. The APOE2 variant is possibly protective against Alzheimer's, but is rare (found in approximately 5% of the population), while the APOE4 variant increases the risk (found in around 25% of the population).

If we think about the diagram above, the combination of alleles for two parents who are both 3/4 is:

Mum

	3	4
3	3/3	3/4
4	3/4	4/4

Dad

In rough terms:

APOE 3/3 means there is no increased risk of Alzheimer's disease.

APOE 3/4 means there is six times the risk, while

APOE 4/4 means there is fifteen times the risk.

These numbers may sound worrying, but it's not all bad news. Remember earlier we talked about genes loading the gun but your environment pulling the trigger? This means having a particular gene does not necessarily mean that it will have an effect; it depends on what 'collides with it' in terms of environment and behaviours. This is known as epigenetics.

On a molecular level, the trigger for Alzheimer's is when amyloid precursor protein (APP) becomes activated and starts to encourage amyloid protein accumulation in the brain. Amyloid in the brain is actually harmless until this activation occurs. In fact, many of us will have beta-amyloid in the brain, which is there to take on functions like regulating nerve function.

So, what actually triggers this process?

If we zoom right in for one moment, the essence of Alzheimer's is when there is a total imbalance between the number of neuronal connections (called synapses) in the brain. It is linked to the way in which the APP molecule gets 'cleaved' (or in simple terms broken down into smaller parts). If APP is cleaved appropriately, it helps to maintain healthy brain function. If not, it leads to a continued build-up of beta-amyloid, which essentially ends up making more of itself, forming clumps and then plaques between neurons affecting connections between them. This aggregation of beta-amyloid is the hallmark of Alzheimer's disease.

Let's just zoom out for a minute to see what this means for us as individuals. In one sense, if we want to prevent or delay Alzheimer's as much as possible, we need to do everything we can to stop the accumulation of beta-amyloid. What does this mean in real life? Does it relate to our typical day, our medical history, or other aspects of the **Health Loop**? Is it to do with our habits and our **How, What and When?**

The answer is: it's all of these.

The 'makers and breakers' of Alzheimer's disease beyond genes [66]

Encourages Alzheimer's disease	Inhibits Alzheimer's disease
Type 2 diabetes	Diet low in refined carbs and high in healthy fats
Processed foods	Whole foods
Sedentary living	Regular exercise
Disturbed sleep	Good sleep

High stress	Low stress
Smoking	Curcumin (see page 151)
Alcohol	Vitamin D

It's great to know all of this in relation to Alzheimer's disease and as you will have seen from the case studies so far, we just need to make whatever we do realistic so that we can prevent illness for as long as possible.

Which brings me back to Janine. By this point, you should almost be able to generate her **Lifestyle Prescription** yourself without my having to reveal it.

Clearly, she did not have Alzheimer's disease, but all the same, her brain was not getting what it needed. She was pre-diabetic (diabetes can increase the risk of Alzheimer's disease by up to 65% if not controlled well) and she had a family history of Alzheimer's. It was obvious from her **Health Loop** that we needed to focus on hormones, diet and movement. Janine had never exercised in her life.

Further exploration around this revealed that Janine had had a strict teacher at school who made her feel like she couldn't do sport, so she'd just stopped trying. It is amazing how powerful childhood experiences can be, both positive and negative. As

Janine was lacking confidence in this area, I started her off on my 'Wake up your muscles' exercises, which you'll find on page 180.

Regarding diet, Janine had always loved comfort foods. She realised she was a bit of a 'sugar addict' (her words). Sugary foods offer an immediate feeling of comfort, but as quickly as the sugar levels go up, they eventually come down, and can make you feel like you're crashing. I knew it was not going to be easy. Janine enjoyed her sweet drinks in the day and her treats at night. We were able to link this back to an event in childhood. She recalled her uncle (her dad's brother) dying suddenly when she was about ten. 'There was a lot of mourning,' she told me. Her dad had a big extended family, and a small army of relatives and friends visited her house over a few days.

She found herself eating biscuits, sweets and chocolates with her cousins, and the food seemed to offer comfort in this time of grief, stress and distress. And so that pattern continued.

The combination of these factors made me pretty sure that Janine was a great candidate for the **IDEAL** framework (see page 26).

Using the framework, we agreed that she could try something called 'graded' for exercise. This is where you build up your activity level gradually. She had always fancied running, but never quite understood how people enjoyed it. After she had mastered the morning wake-up routine, I got her to sign up for Couch to 5K, a fantastic NHS app that gradually builds up your running distance, starting with walking.

As for food, I explained that her blood results showed pre-diabetes, and that her sugar hits were causing crashes in her blood glucose. She wasn't sure if she could give up the crisps and chocolate, so we decided to address it by looking at the **How, What and When** of her eating. Initially, we simply changed the timing; I asked her to eat these treats earlier in the day, and to stop eating for the day around three hours before bedtime. This is often known as time-restricted eating, and it meant that she would not be going to bed with a high blood glucose or blood insulin level.

Blood glucose and insulin levels – why they are important

If there is one thing that makes a big difference to long-term health it is being able to control one's blood sugar level (or blood glucose). It may seem like a dull topic, but so many health issues can be related to insulin resistance and type 2 diabetes.

In summary, refined processed carbohydrates, including biscuits, cakes, white pasta, rice and some commercial cereals, spike our blood glucose levels, This is incredibly common (just think about Amelia, Gary and Janine's **Health Loops**). This means two things. Firstly, these foods are pretty satisfying to eat. If you think about a doughnut, the immediate sugar hit releases dopamine in the brain, giving a feeling of comfort, and your blood sugar level comes up rapidly. Unfortunately, that loading of glucose is not good if it happens repeatedly. It's what our monkey brains crave. Carbohydrate foods like this release dopamine and give us that immediate 'hit' of pleasure and comfort.

In a way, it is our own bodies' response to the sugar that damages us, not the sugar itself. Every time the glucose level rises in the blood, the pancreas churns out insulin to bring the levels down. Insulin is an anabolic hormone, meaning that it aids growth – and that means it also helps lay down fat, and drives the growth of tumours. For these reasons, we do not want too much insulin bounding around our bloodstreams.

Forgetting about *what* we eat for a moment, a simple way to stop this from happening is to cut out snacking, and also to not eat dinner too late.

In Janine's case, she wasn't ready to drop her chocolate snack, so I asked her to have it with her dinner. Why? If you look at the graph below, you can see what happens when we snack. Blood glucose levels go up, and subsequently insulin levels rise in response to this.

Undesirable insulin response and its effect on fat

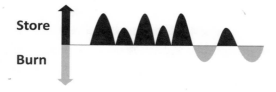

Desirable insulin response and its effect on fat

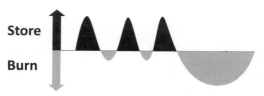

■ Insulin-stimulated fat formation

▨ Fat loss due to reduced insulin

As the graph shows, another effective way of reducing the fat-storing effects of insulin is to not eat for at least twelve hours overnight (unless medically advised otherwise). We sleep for most of this time, so bringing your evening meal forward by an hour or two should be fairly easy. Janine stopped eating three hours before she went to sleep at night, and started to eat breakfast slightly later (while she was at work). Just by doing this, she lost 1.5kg in weight in two weeks without initially changing her diet or activity levels. This does not always work for everyone, and studies give mixed results, but it was very effective in Janine's case, as she is likely to have reduced her glucose and insulin spikes dramatically.

One way of thinking about it is that if we have three meals a day with no snacks in between, we leave a decent gap between our main meals, plus a much longer one overnight when we sleep. This allows our blood glucose and insulin levels to drop appropriately, thereby not encouraging the spikes that eventually lead to 'insulin resistance'. One of the roles of insulin is to take the glucose from the bloodstream and push it into our cells, where we can use it for energy. If there is repeatedly too much glucose in the bloodstream, the insulin levels keep rising in an ineffective attempt to force glucose into the cells. This is insulin resistance, and it can eventually lead to type 2 diabetes.[67] Other conditions associated with insulin resistance include:[68]

- cardiovascular disease

- Alzheimer's disease

- fatty liver

- polycystic ovarian syndrome

- cancer

In Janine's case, after eight weeks, her blood results were significantly improved. She had started running regularly with her children at Parkrun and Junior Parkrun, and she'd also implemented new timings for her meals, stopped snacking and started to eat a low refined-carbohydrate diet. I had warned her about feeling some withdrawal for the first week, and she told me, 'You were right. I felt a bit rough the first week – headaches, plus I was really moody and tired, but after that I started to feel much better.'

She had access to good food at her work canteen. Her breakfast now was usually coffee with eggs or mackerel; for lunch she had a chicken and beetroot or bean salad, and dinner was usually a mound of steamed or roasted veg with olive oil. Janine had also started to use more herbs and spices, like toasted sesame seeds, cumin seeds, rosemary and paprika, to make her food taste more interesting.

Her memory had improved dramatically within three weeks. The brain fog and fatigue had gone, and she felt like she was in the best shape of her life. Her memory loss had been the symptom that scared her into action. 'I just thought I've got to do this for my kids... I need to act now.'

I asked her where she got her comfort fix from now that she'd given up her nightly chocolate treats. Interestingly, she told me she doesn't need any really sweet treats anymore, and actually feels a bit unwell if she has them. She feels more productive and less sluggish, and finds she spends less time planted on the sofa as a result. But Janine and her girls still enjoy a takeaway once a week, and she makes a full-on roast dinner, with Yorkshire pudding, roast potatoes with a glass of wine, at the weekend and it works well for her.

Tweaks

After a few months, we had a chat about making some tweaks to her new lifestyle. Tweaks, which allow a little fine-tuning, are often needed when someone starts to feel better but then wants to feel *even* better. This is a common phenomenon. One tweak that Janine made was to drop the milk and sugar from her coffee. The sugar went first. Initially, she thought she wouldn't be able to hack black coffee, but after a week or so, she started to get used to it. It meant she was leaving out about a pint of milk and six teaspoons of sugar a day without even trying. In addition to this, black coffee is better for us than milky coffee, as the milk attaches itself to the polyphenols (or antioxidants) in the coffee, making them less effective against those free radicals (see page 116).

You may have noticed that I have not come back to the fact that Janine was peri-menopausal. When we first met, she definitely would have been a candidate for prescription hormone replacement therapy (HRT). Although she was not reporting any hot flushes, her brain fog and fatigue were, of course, also common symptoms in peri-menopause. However, the changes she made to her lifestyle are also ones that alleviate symptoms of menopause. Although the increase in her consumption of fish, fruits, nuts and vegetables was directed towards targeting her high blood

135

sugar, her intake of healthy omega-3 fats and other nutrients also have potential benefits in peri-menopause. Omega-3 fats have been shown to potentially ease flushing,[69] and fruit and veg like berries and broccoli contain phyto-oestrogens that increase levels of oestrogen in the body. (Soy, which is well known for this property, is found in miso soup, tofu and soy beans.)

Nuanced self-analysis

The other interesting phenomenon was Janine's own awareness of her eating. She had realised that sweet foods were something she had resorted to after school as a youngster, but it had spiralled out of control. Her mum was brought up in France, where children have an afternoon snack, usually of cake, biscuits or pastries, called *le goûter*. One school of thought is that in France, children do not crave sweet foods during the day, as they know they will be getting something sweet in the afternoon. But if that desire for sweet food spirals out of control, then there is a problem.

Janine also realised that food texture and sound were important to her. She had a thing about quiet eating, and really disliked the noise of chewing and the clattering of knives and forks. She realised she preferred soft foods, like bananas or ripe pears, rather than celery or raw carrots. This was her own **Deep Dive**, if you like. Her own exploration of her relationship with food was revealing, and allowed her to make changes that worked for her.

What Janine needed was gentle encouragement and someone to help her lay out what was going on. Once she had taken stock of her situation, she was able to use the **IDEAL** framework – identify, define, engage, act and look back (see page 26). And that is exactly what she did. As a result, she is likely to feel better for longer, and stave off illness for longer as well.

CHAPTER SUMMARY

- Memory issues are not always related to dementia.

- There are lifestyle interventions that can help prevent the march towards dementia. If left unchecked, type 2 diabetes, peri-menopause and menopause can all be triggers for cognitive decline.

- Blood glucose control and insulin resistance are implicated in many non-communicable diseases.

- Low refined-carbohydrate meals and time-restricted eating, along with good sleep and stress management, can help battle insulin resistance, ease peri-menopause symptoms and help prevent a multitude of diseases.

8

'I WANT TO STOP BEING ILL ALL THE TIME'

Earlier in the book, I mentioned the concept of the **Drawstring Effect**, where we just make one or two small changes, but they seem to tighten up our system rapidly. We also know that sometimes health and illness are finely balanced by an excess of one thing or not getting enough of another.

Sometimes, it can feel like the odds are stacked against you. Illness after illness, followed by ailment after ailment.

I have heard many stories like this over the years, and they can be a real challenge.

I am going to talk about one such case now – this one was a real conundrum.

Johnny was thirty. When he came to see me, he was totally broken. I don't mean broken over a few weeks or months. He told me he had been ill 'all his life'.

He had written his current symptoms down as follows:

- 'always ill'

- IBS

- heartburn

- anxiety

- eczema – never goes

- constant cough and cold

- pins and needles in arms and legs

- neck pain

- cramps

- muzzy head (his words)

- blurred vision

- tinnitus

Before we launch into Johnny's **Health Loop**, it's worth mentioning timelines again.

For really complicated stories, as in the case of Amelia a few chapters ago, I think a timeline is helpful. It's a great exercise to do on yourself. I have often done it with the patient in front of me, and occasionally they will burst into tears once we sit back and stare at it together. The reason for this is because it lays out someone's life and health story in a simple but powerful way. It's also a great adjunct to the **Health Loop**. One is linear, the other not. The subtitle of this book was originally 'Change your health for good by understanding the story of you'. Johnny's story epitomises this.

First off, here is his timeline.

Johnny's timeline

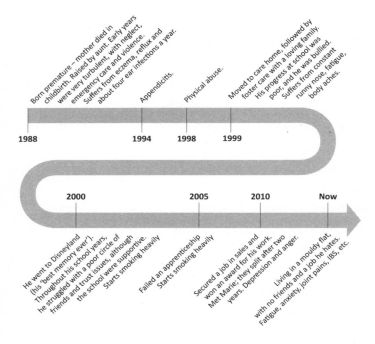

By this stage of the book, I would hope you will immediately be able to see some of the reasons why Johnny finds himself in his current position. It's fair to say that he had had a bad start in life. His biological mother was a single parent with no ties to his birth father. She died in childbirth from a blood clot to her lungs. After a torrid time living at his aunt's house in an environment of domestic abuse, social services placed Johnny in foster care. He was a 'very premature' baby, and was constantly ill for the first few years of life.

The process of healing starts just by looking at the issues and taking stock. Once Johnny saw this timeline drawn out, he became very emotional. It was suddenly obvious why he felt ill all the time.

How do we even start with someone like Johnny? The first thing to understand is that there was going to be no quick fix for him. There were years of trauma there, and too many elements in his story to unpack quickly. What he needed more than anything was compassion and understanding.

Looking at his timeline will tell you that he had gone from being an award-winning sales rep some years ago, to hating his current job (also in sales). Johnny had ended up in sales because he had become good at spinning yarns, talking the talk, as he moved around so much as a child, going from home to home. He also became quite a good liar and social chameleon, enabling him to quickly fit in wherever he went. This made him perfectly suited to the sales role. He had been in some tricky situations as a child and had managed to talk his way out of them. In fact, he'd been so good in his previous job that his boss had given him a bonus that allowed him to buy a flat outright with no mortgage. 'I felt like I was king of the world at that point in my life, but looking back I was lonely and unhappy, living for the next day of sales and partying all night,' he told me. 'I had become addicted to this negative cycle that I couldn't get out of. I became really promiscuous, started acting like an idiot, and was out drinking and smoking every night. I did a bit of cocaine as well. I'd always be the last one out of the bar after a work night out. I was addicted to bad habits but was playing it cool on the outside with a game face, but inside I was dying...'

'OK... what happened after that?'

'Then I met Marie, and things were good for a bit. I was still getting coughs and backache, but drinking through it, basically. She was the love of my life but...' He melted into tears and quickly sniffed himself back into some kind of composure. 'I fucked that up, like I fuck everything up... and she left. She's married now, with a kid.'

'Why do you think you... fucked up?'

'I just kept losing my temper at her for silly things. We just argued all the time... I was a dick.'

'Seems like you have given this a lot of thought. As things are now, what do you think might be worth trying to get you back on to some kind of track?'

'I'm not stupid. I'm lonely. I need to stop drinking, or at least cut down. I've managed to stop smoking, which is one good thing, I guess. I hate work because my boss is a total bully, plus my flat is full of rot and mould after a leak. I need to get that sorted, but I can't be arsed.'

'OK, firstly it's great that you have stopped smoking. What you say all sounds really sensible to me. You mentioned you had eczema and a runny nose all the time. All of the things you mention could be making those symptoms a lot worse, which I am sure you know. Also, your blood pressure is a bit high, which could explain some of the tiredness. That would also come down if you made some changes. Are there any practical things we could start with?'

'I think my flat. I know a plumber who deals with rot and

mould. I don't know whether you can smell it, but it has totally ruined my clothes – and I think that might be making my eczema and runny nose worse. The spray and creams don't really work.'

'OK, that sounds great. What else do you think you could manage at the moment or is that enough for now?'

'I need to get rid of the booze from my house. I'm fine if it's not in the house, but if it is and I'm bored, then that's it – I'll drink it.'

We were basically teasing out the **IDEAL** framework here. He knew what needed to happen, but needed a nudge to help him start.

Johnny's **Health Loop** was obviously telling.

With this kind of story, when the loop tightens, the **Drawstring Effect** (see page 71) can happen quickly, but may be overwhelming. I was cognisant that he was motivated, but he was also quite traumatised from his past. Trauma makes people take on certain behaviours. Johnny had already confessed to arguing with his ex-girlfriend all the time and being a good liar. These are probably results of the survival instincts he would have had to deploy at various points in his life. He had become used to coping with constant upheaval, and occasionally he would look for it – or even inadvertently create it – when it wasn't there.

This is a fairly common pattern in those with significant adverse events. Dr Gabor Maté describes it as the trauma–pain–addiction cycle, where the word 'addiction' can mean a substance or a particular set of behaviours.[70] Unfortunately, these behaviours can be quite destructive once they are not needed day to day. The monkey brain quickly takes over and creates feelings of anger and frustration, meaning any trigger can lead to an impulsive bad behaviour. Remember, the monkey brain is after a short-term hit or fix.

The multitude of issues in Johnny's **Health Loop** does not need writing out. A hard start in life, abuse, rejection, loneliness, heartbreak – that's more than enough to derail someone and lead them towards certain choices and behaviours that then become habits.

Johnny managed to action what he wanted to, and gradually started to get his life back on track. He had generated his own **Lifestyle Prescription**, and by revisiting it every few months with the help of a coach, he managed to work through a lot of issues. There is still a long way to go, but he is well on the way.

CHAPTER SUMMARY

- Early life events have a bearing on our health later in life.

- Adult behaviours can be related to early life trauma.

- Basic needs should be addressed first.

8

'I JUST WANT TO FEEL LIKE I USED TO'

COVID-19 has changed the world. During the pandemic, the world had to come together to fight an enemy that had previously only really existed theoretically, in movies like *Outbreak*, but was always a fearful possibility. At the time of writing, we have had 6.3 million deaths and counting, and there are probably several hundred million people with long COVID.

Despite taking every preventive precaution, following all the medical advice to a tee, there are a group of people who contract COVID and seem to make slow – if any – progress towards recovery. They are often afflicted with multiple symptoms and are given the diagnosis of long COVID.

I am going to tell you about Martha, who is seventy-one. She was a retired librarian who had caught COVID in August 2020. She experienced COVID as a bad flu-like illness, but was just not recovering after several weeks. She had been given steroids and antibiotics by a doctor, but they did not help. She remained breathless for about a month, and then continued to have overwhelming fatigue, brain fog, muscle cramps and palpitations, and found she could hardly exercise.

The main thing that struck me when listening to Martha was that she was grieving for her former life. She had relished her retirement and was heavily involved in her community. She was a regular church attender, played bridge on Tuesday nights and volunteered at a charity shop twice a week. Once a week, her great-nephew and niece would visit her. But that all stopped when COVID came along.

The impact of isolation during lockdown was hard. We know how bad loneliness is for human beings,[71] but the sudden and bizarre nature of the changes enforced by lockdown made it even harder to bear. All of Martha's activities ground to a halt, and she was cut off socially from almost everyone she knew, relying on ad-hoc phone contact. She lived next door to a small supermarket who would drop essentials round, so was able to subsist, but the joy in her life had gone long before her illness came. All she wanted now was to return to her old state of health, but she had been languishing in a 'not well' state for over a year.

Her health story was simple in that she had enjoyed near-perfect health and hardly a sick day in her life, apart from when she was in her mid-forties, when a severe bout of glandular fever had laid her up in bed and kept her off work for six weeks. The ensuing fatigue had lasted another eight weeks after this and Martha's doctor at the time had diagnosed her with a post-viral syndrome.

Curiously, in the GP consulting room, many people who have long COVID[72] often have a story of previous glandular fever or some kind of viral-related fatigue. One phenomenon is that viral infections can effectively 'wake up' viruses which we have previously been infected with that had been lying dormant in our immune systems until they are 'reactivated', leading to symptoms like fatigue. These viruses include Epstein-Barr virus (which causes glandular fever), HHV-6, HSV-1 and CMV.[73]

Let's look at Martha's **Health Loop**.

Martha's Health Loop

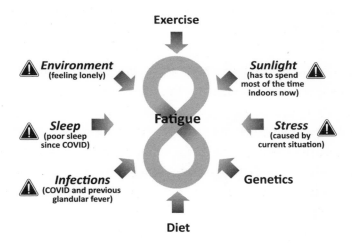

Being a resourceful and determined soul, Martha sought help and advice about long COVID from various news and online resources, as well as her GP, a long COVID clinic in her area, her dentist, her hairdresser, friends at her church group, a local health store and her neighbours, one of whom had become near bedbound with COVID.

She had written a long list of recommendations other people had shared with her (this is her list, not mine, I hasten to add):

- pacing (gradual graded changes in rest and activity):
  - prayer
  - music
  - anti-inflammatory diet

- Medication:
  - steroids
  - antibiotics
  - antivirals

- Supplements:
  - vitamin D – 2,000 units daily
  - vitamin C
  - shilajit
  - turmeric
  - probiotics
  - co-enzyme Q10
  - quercetin
  - omega-3

Out of these, she decided to try everything apart from the medication, as no one was willing to prescribe her these – and, to be fair, if recommended, they would only have been used in the acute phase of COVID, if at all, not several months after the infection.

Martha told me: 'I started pacing and gradually began to do a little more each week, as recommended by the clinic, and I just ordered all the supplements online. I noticed an improvement after just three weeks. I had much better concentration, my brain was working better and I definitely had more energy. I was able to walk up to a mile, after eight weeks of having only managed a few hundred feet. I'd say I am now at about 70% of where I usually am.'

What was going on here? There is actually little evidence for anything that Martha did working effectively on long COVID symptoms, yet Martha clearly felt better. Why? How?

To answer this question, it's probably worth looking at each of the interventions she tried. The first thing is that Martha was really motivated and had good support from her community. She also already had some good healthy habits.

If we think about what Martha did for her own **Lifestyle Prescription**, she gradually increased her activity levels, while at the same time conserving energy. This is one of the tenets of pacing. People with viral or post-viral fatigue run out of energy quickly. Energy comes from the release of the molecule ATP (adenosine triphosphate), which gets broken down to ADP (adenosine diphosphate) within the mitochondria in our cells. I often think of mitochondria as our batteries. People with conditions that lead to long-term fatigue, such as long COVID or fibromyalgia, often have poor mitochondrial function.[74]

To me, an anti-inflammatory diet simply means a diet full of nutrient-rich whole foods, as discussed earlier in the book, and Martha was already eating like this, as she had always been an avid lover of fruits and vegetables high in antioxidants, along with occasional meat and fish. She would often get through a punnet of blueberries in a day.

In terms of prayer, this was something she already practised, and the meditative state achieved during prayer has been shown to be beneficial, as it calms the nervous system via the vagus nerve (which, as we've seen, links the brain to the gut). She also started to listen to relaxing choral music.

What about her stack of supplements? My view on supplements is that they can be beneficial, as long as there is a need for them and you know what is in them.

While we know how they work mechanistically, the evidence around supplements can be patchy. Commercially, supplements form a market worth billions of dollars worldwide, and as such there is often healthy scepticism around their use. There are many people who swear by them, and can even become quite evangelical. Do you have a friend whose life is dominated by turmeric? Or perhaps someone who takes probiotics all the time? I must confess that I used to be a bit like this about vitamin D some twenty years ago – so much so that it became a joke among my colleagues and patients. But at the time, it was because so many people were vitamin D deficient. NICE (the National Institute for Health and Care Excellence) guidance now recommends vitamin D supplementation for many groups.

Vitamin D is well known to have effects on our immunity. Martha's stack of supplements also included vitamin C, which some evidence suggests can reduce oxidative stress and help stave off viruses.

Let's quickly look at the mechanisms of how the other supplements may have been supporting her.

- **Co-enzyme Q10** is an antioxidant found in oily fish that directly supports mitochondria by playing a key role in the electron transfer process, which allows them to function more appropriately. Studies also show that co-enzyme Q10 can support the cardiovascular system.[75]

- **Turmeric** is part of the ginger family, and contains a compound called curcumin that has well-known medicinal properties. Its action is enhanced by piperine (found in black pepper) and has powerful anti-inflammatory and antioxidant effects. For Martha, this may again have helped with a reduction in inflammation and oxidative stress. Studies in animals have shown that turmeric can also boost brain-derived neuro-trophic factor (BDNF), thereby improving brain function.[76][77]

- **Probiotics** are widely available supplemental bacteria that can be consumed to temporarily improve the state of one's gut flora, supporting the microbiome and therefore gut function. They can also help regulate immune responses.[78]

- **Shilajit** is a soil-based supplement containing humic and fulvic acids, which appear to have health benefits in terms of cognition, memory and relieving symptoms of chronic fatigue. It is theorised that it has anti-viral activity thanks to its humic acid component coating viruses, thereby potentially minimising the effects of dormant viruses like HHV-6.[79]

- **Quercetin** is found in coffee, fruits and vegetables and is an antioxidant. Laboratory studies suggest that it can decrease inflammation and allergic responses.[80]

- **Omega-3** is a type of fatty acid with several benefits, including reducing inflammation, helping with anxiety and acting to discourage the stickiness of our blood platelets (platelet clumping can be a feature of long COVID).[81][82]

There is almost no decent grade evidence for any of these supplements when it comes to long COVID specifically – but, as we know, there is never only one thing at play.

The **Drawstring Effect** (see page 71) of the lifestyle changes Martha made, like pacing and tightening up her diet a little, are coupled with several supplements that at least mechanistically could *possibly* have helped reduce inflammation, support mitochondria, knock out free radicals and more. The combination of changes seem to have had pretty good effect in Martha's case.

'Wha'supp?'

Supplements can benefit our health. I take a couple a day myself, but it can be difficult to get good, clear advice on what to take and why; plus, we are all different, and studies do not always account for this. If nothing else, this book will have highlighted that.

Supplements are not without side effects, either, even though they are not prescription medicines. For instance, I have known many people to take too much vitamin C and find it triggers diarrhoea, while excess vitamin D might trigger bone pain, and fish oils could lead to itching. I've also experienced several cases of people taking the wrong version of vitamin B12. Some people may also be taking a supplement that they should really avoid altogether because they are on certain prescribed medications.

In my experience, there has often been a knowledge and accountability gap, which with time needs to be addressed through practitioner education and a conversation between the supplement distributors, scientists, and dietetic, nutrition, pharmacy and medical professionals.

Supplements are sold to the public at most health outlets and supermarkets, but my golden rule is that you cannot supplement your way out of poor health, and you should not take them unless you are convinced there is reason to do so. Patients often ask me where they can find reliable information, advice and evidence on supplements. A good start is www.examine.com/supplements, but the truth is you have to look at the evidence and tailor things to your own needs which is not always easy.

While what she did is not medically recommended, I hope that Martha's case, like those of the others before her, demonstrates the power of laying out the story, honing in on the bits that need tightening up, and then actioning the **Lifestyle Prescription**. In Martha's case she did it all herself, out of sheer desperation, as, at the time of writing, medical support has not yet caught up with the demands of long COVID. Clinical research on microclots in the blood and the effects of reactivated viruses in terms of the dysfunctional effects on the autonomic nervous system continue.

CHAPTER SUMMARY

- Long COVID can be highly debilitating and affects many biological systems, giving rise to symptoms that reflect immune dysfunction.

- Pacing can be a useful tool for recovery from fatigue.

- Fatigue can suggest mitochondrial dysfunction, but in long COVID it can also be down to poor blood flow from platelet clumping.

- Supplements can potentially be a useful adjunct to lifestyle change.

III

8

THE FIXES

"You have to go the way your blood beats."
James Baldwin

8

PUTTING IT ALTOGETHER

There are so many variables with illness. The cases you have read so far will, by now, have given you a good flavour of the variety of things that collude to affect our health. Now, I want to slow down, reflect, and take a good look at why we should bother with our health in the first place. My GP trainer, Ed Peile, used to do a tutorial where he would simply ask:

'What's the point?'

It is easy in the current climate to just think, 'Sod it, you know what? Life is short. I'm gonna do whatever the heck I like.' And truth be told, that was me from the age of fourteen until the age of about thirty. But lives and times change. Stuff happens to us as the years go by, and as time goes on, we have to work harder at things that we used to take for granted.

That's probably a good rule for life – take nothing for granted.

If you have ever seen someone who has difficulty doing the simplest things, like walking a few steps, getting out of a chair or picking up a cup to drink, as a result of physical or mental illness, then you will understand how hard life can be.

Several years ago, when I was still doing some work in broadcasting, I got some insight into this. I had to wear some goggles that mimicked a severe eye condition, making me partially sighted (almost blind). It was hugely distressing. After a few minutes, I felt frustrated, agitated and impatient. But most of all, I was scared. It was genuinely uncomfortable, even though I knew I could take the goggles off at any time. It really made me understand more about what life must be like for someone with partial sight, albeit briefly.

Some years later, at City University, I tried on an empathy suit that mimicked a stroke. I was strapped up into a suit which made it impossible to move one side of my body. They then put on a pair of electrically charged gloves that mimicked neuropathy pain (agonising at higher settings), and those goggles again. This is used as a training tool for nursing students, so that they can really relate to their patients, and I could see how effective it could be. Once again, that experience really stayed with me.

My point is that if illness strikes, then so be it, but if there is a way of us enjoying a good quality of life, free of pain and distress for as long as possible, then we should really strive for that, grab it, and savour every minute of the journey while we are at it.

It's not all good vs bad

Several years ago, I met a friend for dinner in London. He lives in a scenic part of Asia and his home affords stunning views. He was telling me about his morning routine, which involved waking up at 5am, stretching, drinking fresh water and then going for a run. He would then come back, do ten minutes of meditation or yoga, and then (you will never guess what comes next)... he smokes a cigarette.

It was like a record scratch moment. I just wasn't expecting him to say that. It really made me think.

While I would never encourage anyone to take up smoking, his experience is quite different to someone nipping out of the office for a quick power-puffed rushed cigarette in the rain. He sits quietly on a veranda and looks out over the desert. And he smokes just that one cigarette a day. Clearly, the cigarettes are doing him some harm, and I did ask him, given his incredibly mindful morning routine, why he didn't just try to simply mimic the breathing pattern he uses when smoking a cigarette.

What he was doing, though, was savouring the moment, albeit with something that is clearly unhealthy. But on balance, given the rest of his routine, his **Health Loop** could be a lot worse.

Although this is a 'bad' example, I find that savouring is a good thing to remember. Really *savour* whatever it is you are doing: the taste of your tea, being with your friends, swimming in the sea. Just being in the moment is a great way to mindfully proceed in life. It stops the mind from wandering and allows one to be present.

Prepare for the unpredictable — that's life

You now know how to set yourself up for success. In essence, you take stock by using the **Health Loop**, which generates a **Lifestyle Prescription**, while the **IDEAL** framework helps you to activate and live out the behaviours you need to see change.

But as we know, life is complex, and we often get sideswiped by events such as day-to-day stresses, bereavement, emergencies and unforeseen problems. Sometimes, life does its best to derail us. It can be hard not to resort to bad habits when this happens.

We often seek comfort to relieve emotional pain. The tough part is sitting with that pain, wherever it comes from, and working through it. This has never been more relevant than in the times we are living through right now, wherever you are in the world.

There is no easy way around this, but a rule of thumb is to use any method that does not harm yourself or others to get through it, whether that means reading, meditating, talking to friends or prayer. My own favourite method is to really be present and savour everything that is good, by really living in the moment and letting negative thoughts pass through in a flash without holding on to them, however hard things might be. This means doing things like really tasting each mouthful of odd or clocking the eye colour of the person you are talking to – truly paying attention and being present.

Be aware of your inner monkey and the way it can make you react without thinking. Remember to check yourself. The monkey brain is irrational and impulsive; as much as it can sometimes help you to have fun, it can also hijack your grown-up brain when the chips are down, leading you back into a spiral of bad behaviours. Be aware of your monkey; be kind to it, and only allow it out when appropriate!

Start by focusing on yourself

At the beginning of this book, I talked about behaviours. These are key, but even if you have already dived in and started making changes, I still want you to take a moment now and really think about yourself. What will ultimately keep you on track is your mindset, your grounded habits, your self-belief and your compassion towards yourself.

Before embarking on your **Health Fix** journey, it's a good idea to work out what your values are, what your purpose might be, and how you can grow emotionally and spiritually. I first did this about twenty years ago, and it was a revelation.

Although many coaches say you cannot easily coach yourself, if you could, this is not a bad start.

Try to identify your core values, which will ultimately reveal what drives you as a person.

Pick or tick as many words as you like that relate to you and your values from the list below.

abundance	cheerfulness	empathy
acceptance	cleverness	encouragement
accountability	collaboration	enthusiasm
achievement	commitment	ethics
adventure	community	excellence
advocacy	compassion	expressiveness
ambition	competitiveness	fairness
appreciation	consistency	family
attractiveness	contribution	flexibility
autonomy	co-operation	freedom
balance	creativity	friendships
benevolence	credibility	fun
boldness	curiosity	generosity
brilliance	daring	grace
calmness	decisiveness	growth
caring	dedication	happiness
challenge	dependability	health
charity	diversity	honesty

humility
humour
inclusiveness
independence
individuality
innovation
inspiration
intelligence
intuition
joy
kindness
knowledge
leadership
learning
love
loyalty
mindfulness
motivation
open-mindedness
optimism
originality
passion
peace

perfection
performance
personal development
playfulness
popularity
power
practical
preparedness
proactive
proactivity
professionalism
punctuality
purposefulness
quality
recognition
relationships
reliability
resilience
resourcefulness
responsibility
responsiveness
risk-taking
safety

security
self-control
selflessness
service
simplicity
spirituality
stability
success
teamwork
thankfulness
thoughtfulness
tradition
trustworthiness
understanding
uniqueness
usefulness
versatility
vision
warmth
wealth
well-being
wisdom

Once you have done that, group together similar words in four columns, e.g.:

cleverness	reliability	health	charity
Intelligence	consistency dependability honesty	wellbeing joy	contribution

161

Then pick one word from each as the main word in each column:

cleverness	reliability	health	charity
intelligence	**consistency** dependability honesty	**wellbeing** joy	contribution

Lastly, to crystallise these, write a sentence with each one that applies to you. For example:

I will use my intelligence to help others at work.
Consistency is important in my family life.
I want to encourage wellbeing.
Contribution is a part of everything I do.

Next, grab a pen and a pad and write down the answers to the following questions:

1. What do others consistently say about me?
   (This gives you a clue about your behaviours.)

2. Who or what are negative or toxic forces in my life?
   (These you will need to remove or avoid.)

3. Who or what are the positive forces in my life?
   (These are your support slings. Look after them.)

4. What am I deeply interested in and what do I love to do?
   (These will give you some focus.)

The Health Fix toolkit

In order to use this final section of the book, here is a summary of your *Health Fix* toolkit:

1. Understand your behaviours

2. Be aware of your monkey brain

3. Symptoms relate to systems

4. Understand your **Health Loop**

5. Remember the **IDEAL** framework

6. Embrace your **Lifestyle Prescription**

7. Repeat the process as often as you like

I am going to split the rest of this section into different parts of the **Health Loop**, as we know that they are all factors that affect our health. We will be focusing on diet, exercise, sleep and stress, as these are the areas where you can make changes, but it can be hard to know where to start. You cannot alter your genes or change your history of infections but awareness of them means that you can focus on the other elements of your **Health Loop** to mitigate the impact they may have on you.

The previous chapters should have left you with a fairly good understanding of most of what makes up your 'source code'. Now it is time to push the buttons and execute it all.

Things will start to click into place as you start to see the interconnectedness of the **Health Loop**. One of my patients, Anna, looked at the sunlight part of her **Health Loop** after being found to have vitamin D deficiency. She realised her mum and brother both had vitamin D deficiency too, after asking them about it, despite their living in a hot, sunny part of Europe. Anna had an office job, lived in the UK and spent little time outdoors, but after making an effort to go out more and taking a vitamin D supplement regularly, her levels came up nicely and she felt far less tired.

She realised that her deficiency could be a combination of both her genes and a lack of sunlight – both elements of the **Health Loop**. We do not know for sure, but it is possible that her family has a VDR gene variation. One in four people have a form of this gene 'mutation', meaning they cannot effectively activate vitamin D, so often need higher doses. In my own clinical practice, I find these are the group who are often already supplementing with vitamin D and getting sun exposure, but their levels are persistently low.

The point is that whatever angle we look at this issue from, whether we focus on the genetic part or the sunlight, the **Health Loop** will lay things out for you and usually reveal an answer.

Feeling worse before you feel better

Many of my patients over the years have reported feeling a bit rough when they first start any kind of health kick or improvement. This is completely natural and often associated with withdrawal, especially when changing diet, for instance cutting down on processed foods, caffeine, sugar or alcohol.

Commonly, people report feelings of fatigue and headaches, but rest assured it will pass, usually within a week. The same can happen when you start exercising for the first time. Support yourself by staying well hydrated, keep moving and prioritise your sleep. Remember, it is only temporary and in a few days' time you are likely to feel far better than you did before.

Start and end the day the right way – the power of a mindful minute

There are a few things worth doing at the beginning and end of each day if you can fit them in. It's mainly about checking in on how you feel in your body and mind. You might have some kind of stressful thought bounding around in your head; you might feel tense; you might feel great.

In the morning, if you are busy, then it's all rush, rush, rush. But most things can wait for one minute.

When you first open your eyes, just allow yourself to come to terms with the new day. Sit at the edge of your bed and think about how you feel – physically and mentally. Sit on the side of your bed and gently stand up. Take note of how you feel.

Shortly, you will see my favourite wake-up routine ('Wake up your muscles each morning', see page 180), which I highly recommend, but if I am feeling tense or worried about something, I will also tend to do an indulgent one-minute recharge (see page 67) with belly breathing (see page 178). Often, I will do it while imagining that I am lying on a beach. Sometimes, it's so vivid that I swear I can actually feel the warmth of the sun I am imagining on my face – it's amazing how powerful the mind can be.

In any case, it can set you up well for the day. As I mentioned earlier, I also do this one-minute recharge in my car when I pull up at work and again when I arrive home. Many people who struggle with anxiety have found this easy-to-fit-in recharge helpful.

What about the very end of the day, in terms of our minds? My patient Robin once shared his end-of-day ritual with me. He uses it to make sure that anything that has been bothering him from that day is set aside in his mind before he sleeps. He closes his eyes, focuses on the problems or issues, and accepts that there are many things he cannot solve or are out of his control. It's almost like the one-minute recharge, but it's about letting go of the angst around the problems that the world has thrown at you that day.

Doing this helps him sleep without worrying, meaning he literally never 'loses sleep over stuff'. We will look at sleep more closely on pages 190–194, but this idea of resolution or acceptance is a simple idea, and I have found that it really helps, particularly in people who tend to 'overthink' or are perfectionists and may find it hard to switch off.

Exploring the Fixes

OK, so now it is time to give you a load of quick tips. I understand that life is busy and complex, so I preface all of my 'tips' in the coming pages with the words *'whenever possible...'*

At the start of the book, I explained that to make this work for you, it was not just a case of rushing to the 'Fixes' section at the back. This whole book is a toolkit that makes much more sense now that you have taken the time to understand the *Health Fix* journey.

By now, you may well have a clear idea of your own **Health Loop**. You may even have started on your *Health Fix* journey. The tips and tools that follow are there to really supercharge your journey and make things even easier for you. There are also some basic daily prevention hacks to avoid some common modern pitfalls that can lead to symptoms.

8

DIET

Remember, there is no such thing as the 'best' diet. Your diet is individual to you. **How, What and When** you eat is also down to you. That said, there are some principles worth following, and these are captured below. You have read enough in the patient stories now to understand the nuances.

The mission is simple in some ways: eat for pleasure, for energy, to nourish your immune system and to keep you well.

Now, here are some generic tips.

How to eat

- Chew your food slowly and don't take the next mouthful until after the first one has reached your stomach.

- Savour and really taste each mouthful.

- Sit while you are eating.

- Eat quietly away from screens (eat mindfully).

- If enjoying a side salad, then eat it before your main meal (this helps to control blood glucose spikes).

- Bake or steam your main meals if you can.

- Drink water regularly throughout the day inbetween meals.

What to eat

- A glass of fresh water first thing in the morning with any supplements or medication.

- A wide variety of whole foods that are not processed – 'eat the rainbow', as many people like to say.

- Plenty of high-fibre foods, like fruits, nuts and vegetables, including a portion of green vegetables every day.

SMOOTHIE TIME

If you struggle to get fruits and vegetables into your diet, then think about storing a load in your freezer compartment and enjoying them blended as a smoothie for breakfast. If you have a smoothie blender, this is a quick way to get a hit of nutrients.

(My own smoothie is a little different each day, depending on what is left in the freezer, but it usually contains celery, spinach, ginger, beetroot, mixed berries, half a banana, walnuts, coconut yogurt and water. My colleagues at work are used to me walking down the corridor to the fridge where I store this delicious gloop, which I slurp for breakfast at around 10am.)

NUTRIENT-RICH FOODS

There is no such thing as a 'superfood', but there are certain foods that are high in nutrients including:

- leafy greens, like kale, spinach and watercress

- broccoli, cauliflower, cabbage, Brussels sprouts, asparagus

- peppers

- carrots and parsnips

- garlic

- parsley, coriander, basil and other fresh herbs

- berries, like blueberries, raspberries and black-berries

- beetroot

- wild salmon, mackerel and sardines (omega-3)

- flaxseeds, walnuts, seaweed, algae, chia seeds (vegan omega-3)

- beef

- liver

- green beans

- eggs

- lentils

- artichokes

- avocado

- tomatoes

- mushrooms

- sweet potatoes

If you feel any of these foods are having a bad effect on you after you eat them, remember you can try a four-week elimination as explained on page 92.

THE QUEEN OF OILS

Extra virgin olive oil is my staple oil of choice.[83] It has benefits for the cardiovascular system, but truth be told, it is just freely available to buy and tends to go with all types of cooking, as well as making a great dressing, and that's really why I am such a fan. It also tastes naturally sweet. There are, of course, many other oils that can be of benefit to us in terms of reducing inflammation, including avocado, walnut, grapeseed, sesame and coconut oils, but extra virgin olive oil gets the crown in my eyes.

Note: The benefits of an oil depend on its smoke point (the higher the better), as it will tend not to produce the harmful free radicals that I mentioned on page 116, unlike oils with a low smoke point.

HERBS AND SPICES:
PLANT-POWERED 'MEDICINE'

Herbs and spices have numerous potential health benefits. Most of us know about the anti-inflammatory properties of many of these from science articles, websites and magazines.

It's hard to get these into your diet unless you can cook with them, so I personally use the first three on the list on the next page in my morning smoothie, and most of the rest in basic cooking – whether that be with extra virgin olive oil and vegetables, or on a chicken with roast potatoes and some rosemary. It does not have to be complicated.

They are worth incorporating, not only because they are usually rather tasty, but also for that power of marginal gains I mentioned at the beginning of the book (see page 28). Remember your imaginary identical twin from earlier? Well, if you eat anti-inflammatory foods most days, and your twin eats processed foods on most days, then there is likely to be a difference in how you both feel, and possibly also in your long-term health outcomes.

Here are my favourite herbs and spices:

- cinnamon – helps control blood glucose[84]

- ginger – anti-inflammatory

- turmeric – anti-inflammatory[85]

- garlic (raw is best) – anti-inflammatory, antiviral and lowers blood pressure[86]

- black pepper – anti-inflammatory[87]

- rosemary – anti-inflammatory, antioxidant-rich and helps control blood glucose[88]

- sage – antioxidant-rich[89]

- basil – supports immune function[90]

There are plenty more herbs not covered here that can also have medicinal effects, but if you can incorporate just the ones listed here into your week, you will be doing well. A good tip for those who need help with blood glucose control is to add standard vinegar to savoury foods. This will help to reduce spikes in blood glucose by slowing down the breakdown of carbohydrates.

DRINK UP

Water – The most important thing in any diet is water. Unless advised otherwise, two litres a day, including a glass after you wake up in the morning, is good to aim for. (There is a lot of debate about the quality of tap water, but filters can be prohibitively expensive.)

Tea and coffee – Teas (black, silver or green) and coffee are far more beneficial in terms of antioxidant power if taken *without* milk.[91]

In terms of your genes, you may be a fast or slow caffeine metaboliser. If you feel jittery after a coffee, you probably metabolise it slowly, and it may be better for you to have drinks without caffeine. My own favourite is green rooibos tea. Drink all your caffeine before midday to aid sleep at night.

Alcohol – If you happen to drink alcohol, then red wine and whisky[92] (in moderation) are favoured. Both are rich in polyphenols, which can protect the heart and also help diversify the gut microbiome – which, as we know, nourishes the immune system.

When to eat

- Eat main meals at regular intervals (or when you feel hungry), with no snacks in between, as they spike blood glucose.

- Drink water after a meal and throughout the day, not just during a meal, as this can spike blood glucose. If you find drinking water hard work, then perhaps add some berries, lemon, lime, cucumber or rosemary to change the taste.

- Eat dinner, unless advised otherwise, around three hours before you go to bed, with no snacking afterwards.

- If you wake up and generally do not feel hungry, then drink water, black or green tea or black coffee, and have breakfast a little later.

- Stop eating when you feel full.

- If you fancy something sweet as a treat, it is best to eat it straight after a meal to reduce the spike in blood glucose.

- Walk for 10 minutes after a meal to reduce the spike in blood glucose.

CHAPTER SUMMARY

- Eat a variety of whole foods.

- Eat dinner early rather than late.

- Stay well hydrated.

- Food diaries can be helpful.

8

EXERCISE: MOVEMENT AND POSTURE

The way we move as human beings has changed in the last thousand years. Most of us no longer need to pick fruit from trees, roll logs, use spears or swim outdoors. So we need to make sure we deliberately 'wake up' various muscle groups to ensure that they 'fire' properly.

Activate ➡ Stretch ➡ Strengthen ➡ Keep Moving

Whatever you do during the day that is excessive, however necessary it may be for work or another reason, whether that's sitting and reading, writing on a laptop at a desk or lifting boxes in a factory, there needs to be some kind of counterbalance.

If you sit for hours at a desk, you need to stand and stretch for one maybe two minutes every hour – or you may wish to invest in a sit-stand desk. We have these at my surgery, and the evidence shows that standing up at a desk bestows many benefits on our health, including the cardiovascular system, as well as improving engagement at work.[93] In fact, just sitting up and moving around briefly every ten minutes has huge benefits for our metabolism in terms of preventing conditions like diabetes. I experienced this first-hand myself when I moved to a different GP practice. I used to push a button to summon patients in my old surgery and at the new one I was moving to the waiting room every ten minutes. Within a year, I had unintentionally dropped 10kg in weight with no change to any of my other habits.

The other reason to keep moving is to make sure you retain muscle mass as you age. Sarcopenia is the loss of muscle mass as we age and is a significant risk to our health.[94]

If you find that you are hunched over a computer, then do pay attention to your posture and screen height. These are basic things, of which most of us are aware.

Our upright posture should be head up, shoulders relaxed and core tummy muscles working (for the latter, imagine a spring running from your belly button back through to your back and keep it nice and taut).

Beyond this, as mentioned before, it is important to 'wake up' or charge groups of muscles so that they fire appropriately. Doing this will prevent stiffness, enable you to move more easily and improve your sense of vitality.

Based on common medical complaints I see in my practice, two of the biggest problem areas for desk-based workers are breathing and the pelvis. We will explore breathing further now, while the 'Wake up your muscles' exercise on page 180 can pay huge dividends.[95]

Breathing

Most people do not see breathing as a form of 'exercise', yet poor breathing technique can lead to anxiety, chest pain, fatigue and insomnia – and vice versa. It's a two-way street, so these issues can also impact breathing.

BELLY BREATHING

There are so many wonderful breathing exercises that can help relax us, but if I had to pick one to master in terms of long-term health it would be diaphragmatic breathing, a technique often used by singers.

This is essentially what is known as belly breathing. You want to be able to breathe in and out smoothly through your nose (or your mouth, if you really prefer) *without* your shoulders rising and falling, and *without* your chest moving in and out. Your belly will move, but not your chest. This encourages proper gaseous exchange in the deepest parts of your airways.

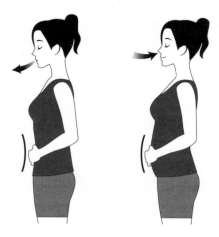

Sit down, place one hand on your chest and one on your belly, and breathe in and out slowly. Allow your belly to move, but not your chest.

This technique makes your diaphragm go up and down, while strengthening our core abdominal muscles. It aids relaxation and improves oxygen intake.

Slow, deep diaphragmatic breathing also stimulates the vagus nerve, which will help with your sense of calm and relaxation, as described on page 67.

For most people, breathing offers a really palpable connection between the mind and body. Just think about the number of times you have sighed or gasped because of something on your mind. It is the one function that truly binds the mental and physical consciously, yet most of us do it totally subconsciously. Unless there is a problem with our breathing, we tend to breathe without thinking too much about it.

Movement

What about the way we move the rest of our muscles? What works? Do we need to be running every day? Is yoga better than Pilates? Is swimming good or bad for your back? These questions often dominate our minds, and for me there are no hard and fast rules, just some principles. This is because everyone is different.

Unless extreme, pretty much any movement or exercise is good for us but working out which type is right for us can be useful. I think the exercise on the next page is a good place to begin.

Wake up your muscles each morning

The first rule of exercise is to make sure that your muscles are ready to 'fire'. This is something that is often overlooked. It's the step before stretching. If you ever get that stiff or slow feeling in the morning, or feel like your legs are tired by the time you have got to the top of a set of stairs, then this exercise will really help you. It also addresses two key anatomical areas: the chest, for breathing, and the movement of the hips and pelvis.

First things first. How we start our day is all important. When you wake up in the morning, calibrate yourself by gently moving from sitting on the edge of the bed to see how you feel. It feels a little different day to day, but may not be something you actively take notice of.

Next, get into the right frame of mind. Focus on something that makes you feel good (imagine sitting on a beach, thinking of time spent with your best friends, or a memory of yourself or your favourite footballer scoring a winning goal). This positive framing of mind is really important. When you are ready, do the following:

Massage either side of your sternum and ribs in small, firm circles, moving along the side of your breastbone and down the edge of the ribcage, in the path as shown in the top diagram, opposite, for around two minutes. Belly-breathe continuously as you do this, and feel how your chest feels less tense by the end. The massaging may feel a little uncomfortable at first, but this is to be expected.

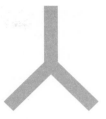

Sit on the side of your bed or on a chair and massage your lower abdomen in circles to wake up your psoas muscle (the large muscle, blacked out in the diagram below*, which helps you raise your thighs towards your belly button while standing, or what is otherwise known as hip to trunk flexion). Aim for the points halfway between your hip bone and belly button, and massage massage simultaneously in quite firm circles for one minute.

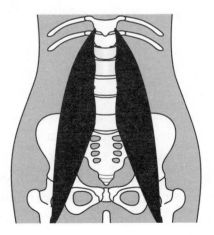

* You cannot actually access or directly feel the psoas muscle through the front of the abdomen, but the pressure helps to activate it.

Do the half or full pigeon pose stretch shown in the diagram below to help fire your gluteal muscles. Do this for one minute on each side.

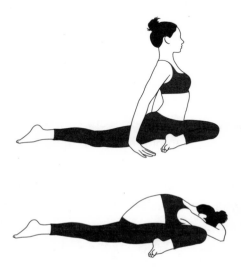

Now, how do you feel?

To feel the immediate effects of this 'waking up' exercise, sit down and stand up again from your sitting position, or perhaps walk up some stairs to see how much easier it feels than normal.

This is a great practice to start each day. Always remember to start in the right frame of mind, and if you cannot do it in the mornings because life is too busy, then any time of day will do. I sometimes spread these exercises out, but they are best done in one go.

Types of exercise

The bottom line is that in order to stay healthy, we need to try to do as many of these types of exercise as we can:

- strength

- balance

- flexibility

- endurance

The key is to work out what kind of movement suits you best. Each person reading this will have a different regime. You may be someone who runs every week in a group, or cycles, or swims – or you may not do anything yet. It matters not. Movement and exercise should, above all, be safe – and, ideally, fun.

I have come across many cases of dubious techniques with sports that have led to back and joint pains and have required the help of skilled physical therapists to put right. I have also come across people whose way of doing things has led to such pains, such as people sleeping on their front, which puts strain on the lower back and can cause carpal tunnel syndrome symptoms (pins and needles in the forearm and hand) from sleeping with their forearms compressed by a pillow.

And how many of us get bad backs from not using our knees when bending down to pick something up off the floor or lifting something heavy? The number of manual workers or parents of toddlers I see with bad backs from constant bending is staggering.

If you are new to the world of exercise, then take things slowly. There is an element of 'no pain, no gain' in that if you have not moved regularly in a while, you will need some time to get used to it like Janine did. It gets easier, and it will enrich your life. You will feel more energised and more mobile. Start small, if you like – even one star jump a day will have some benefit.

Many people already know the benefits of going to the gym, training in a martial art or even archery (where breath control is key), but you can start with something simpler, like walking or cycling.

If you are a newbie, or returning to exercise after a long break, remember you might feel worse before you feel better. Don't be put off! Many people who exercise for the first time often find that they need to have a nap afterwards or lie down on the sofa. This is because they are not used to that level of energy expenditure and their mitochondria (the tiny organs within the cells that produce our energy), are working overtime. This passes as time goes on and exercise tolerance builds up.

STRENGTH

If you are looking for an easy way to start, then for strength you can push off the walls, do gentle squats or use dumbbells or weights. (As I am writing this at home, I can see my dumbbell under my desk, and I occasionally stop and do a few bicep curls – usually six, sometimes twelve. This works for me. It is accessible and easy, and so I do it.)

BALANCE

For balance, you can do anything from 'walking the log' in the park or standing on one leg with your eyes closed (be careful with this, as it is harder than it looks). You could also do one-leg side lifts, walk in a straight line going from heel to toe, as if you were walking a tight rope (for a bigger challenge, do it with your eyes closed), or, if you have a gym ball, you can sit on that.

A harder balance exercise is to stand on one leg, then bend down and pretend to pick up an imaginary sock off the floor, then put it on the foot that is off the ground.

Walking

For most people, the easiest exercise that can cover strength, balance, flexibility and endurance is walking. For instance, on a long muddy walk over uneven terrain where you have to watch your step, you really have to use your balance. And if you plan a route that's about ten kilometres long, it is likely to do you a world of good in terms of all four types of exercise. I love a long walk, and prefer it to running. I speed up and slow down when I want to. Although I personally do not generally run long distances, I do tend to run or rush everywhere, whether it is a quick burst up the stairs at work or a speedy dash to the grocer's around the corner.

The Tarahumara peoples from Mexico[96] are famed for being able to run hundreds of miles, because as a community they run much of the time, scampering everywhere with quick, light steps on their forefeet rather than their heels. Part of the Tarahumara's ethos is to run with 'contagious joy'.

Invisible 'exercise'

Habitual exercise, whether it's the constant running of the Tara-humaras or the fact that some people, including myself, tend to jog up the stairs, bestows a person with high 'NEAT' (non-exercise activity thermogenesis).[97] This basically means you burn off calories just by virtue of the way you get through the day, expending energy through random background daily activities, like jiggling your legs under the table or climbing the stairs.

Just look at the diagram below to see how many calories we burn through NEAT – almost double what we do from formal exercise. A common way of exploiting this is to use a standing desk in the office. It cuts down your sitting time and allows you to exercise lightly without really noticing it.

NEAT is often a key difference between the person who 'cannot sit still' and the person who literally does not move a muscle when sitting down.

Total calorie consumption

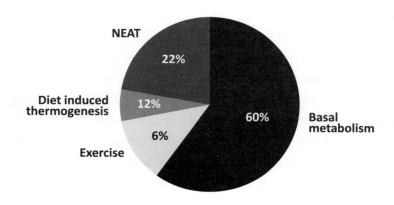

What feels right for you?
Do the doable and build on it

We know that movement and exercise have multiple benefits – that's old news.

When it comes to the actual exercise part of the diagram opposite, it's all about what you like doing and what works for you. Exercise is a key part of the **Health Loop**, but you can tailor it to suit your needs. If you are a highly strung person who runs on adrenaline, then you may wish to choose something more calming, like strength work or yoga, rather than doing a load of aerobic exercise that may actually increase your adrenaline output and raise your blood pressure.

I used to do yoga regularly. I found the first few weeks hard, but I felt so invigorated and 'more alive' after a few sessions that it quickly became a habit. It all stopped with the pandemic, and I am keen to restart my yoga classes as I write. It was definitely the right type of exercise for me.

If you are like Janine and you simply need to make a start, then brisk walking is a great place to begin. Walk for half an hour a day if you have time; if not, then just walk as much as you can.

What works best for me is a combination of quick HIIT (high intensity interval training) exercises each morning. HIIT exercises are a great option for people who are short on time and want to improve blood glucose control. The whole idea is to get your heart rate up quickly. You only need to do one minute of HIIT each morning and then stretch to relax afterwards, almost as a reward. Some HIIT exercises are illustrated on the next page.

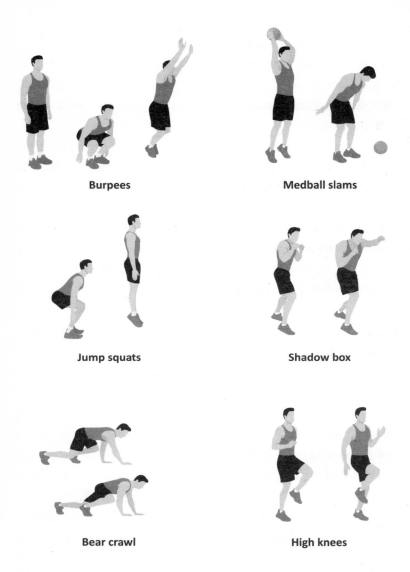

Burpees

Medball slams

Jump squats

Shadow box

Bear crawl

High knees

If you have the time and resources, then it may be worth hiring a personal trainer or exercise coach to work out the best kind of movement for you.

The truth is that the benefits and ease of exercise are cumulative, and the law of marginal gains we covered in the first part of the book (see page 28) plays a powerful role. I find that following the rules around behaviour change makes it much easier to stick with the programme:

- Make it easy (e.g. start with a simple sequence which is quick and fits in to your day with ease)

- Tag it on to an existing behaviour (e.g. just after your morning coffee)

- Say well done to yourself

And for some reason if I don't do it, it matters not. I can do it later in the day, or just resume tomorrow.

CHAPTER SUMMARY

- Move whenever and wherever you can.

- Make it fun.

- Think about the right type of exercise for you.

- Wake up your muscles in the morning.

8

SLEEP

I f there is a function or part of the **Health Loop** that is grossly underestimated, then it's sleep. In today's world, we are often so busy that we fail to prioritise this key physiological function. I have done it myself: you get home at 8.30pm, eat some food and then start to work through other things that need attention. Before you know it, the clock says 1.30am. Sound familiar?

Poor sleep, or lack of good-quality sleep, over a long period leads to illness – end of. That includes type 2 diabetes, heart disease and Alzheimer's disease. It took well over forty years for the penny to drop for me, but the science on this is clear. Sleep gives the body a chance to restore itself in terms of cellular function (known originally as the restorative theory of sleep),[98] so we need to show it some respect and not think of it as a waste of time.

What is your chronotype?

Everything in your body follows a natural rhythm.[99] If you have ever suffered jet-lag or worked night shifts, then you will know what happens to your brain and body when they are out of their natural rhythm. You have probably heard of the circadian rhythm, which in some ways really is the rhythm of life.

The circadian rhythm responds to light and dark, and works as the 'body clock', affecting everything from appetite and blood pressure to concentration and reaction times. There are also what are known as chronotypes. You may have heard people described as owls and larks in the past, but a more helpful way to understand it may be to look at the four classifications below. Do you recognise yourself as one of these?

Understanding chronotypes

Lion
10–20%

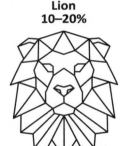

Waketime: 4–7am
Bedtime: 8–9pm
Most productive: Early morning

Bear
50%

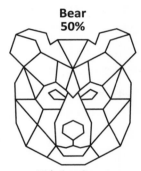

Waketime: Sun-up
Bedtime: Sun-down
Most productive: Late morning

Wolf
10–20%

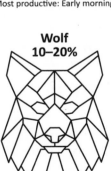

Waketime: 8–10am
Bedtime: 1–2am
Most productive: Mid-day & evening

Dolphin
50%

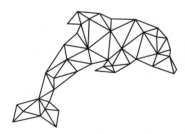

Waketime: Irregular
Bedtime: Irregular
Most productive: Late morning

You will notice that most people are bears.

In a way, what we want is not just to sleep better, but also to be in tune with our own body clocks. If we understand our chronotypes, we can do things while we are awake to improve how we sleep. If you see yourself in one of these chronotypes, then try to adapt your work or day schedule accordingly.

A classic example of this is teenagers. The circadian rhythm changes during and after puberty, and their response to light and dark alters with these hormonal changes. Our natural tendencies are to be wakeful when it is light and sleepy when it is dark.

This is down to melatonin, which is the hormone the brain's pineal gland releases to naturally aid sleep. Melatonin is triggered by darkness, but is released later in teenagers, which means they naturally want to go to bed late, and the knock-on effect is that they then want to sleep in. This is a normal part of adolescence. Imagine if schools changed the timing of their classes and exams to start later in the day to fit in with this: what kind of impact might that have on the performance of their teenage students?

In the same way, think about things you can change in your day that may benefit your chronotype. I have a wolf chronotype, so tend to 'come alive' a little later in the day. Because of this, I prefer to complete more complex tasks in the afternoon, not the morning.

Tips for sleep

Most tips for better sleep are relatively simple, but the truth is, to get good sleep, there are various non-sleep activities that you need to consider. Because of this, you'll notice that the tips I share below are not just about sleep but overlap with other areas in the **Health Loop**.

Realistically speaking, you may not be able to do all of these, but the more you can manage, the better. There are literally hundreds of sleep tips out there, so see what works for you – and obviously start with the basics, like a comfortable mattress and pillow.

- Go to bed at the same time each night and wake up at the same time each morning.

- Stay in bed for approximately eight hours, if you can.

- Expose yourself to natural light first thing in the morning and during daylight hours.

- Avoid caffeine after midday.

- Avoid having alcohol close to bedtime.

- Avoid large meals and drinks close to bedtime.

- Avoid vigorous exercise within two hours of bedtime.

- Avoid blue light (which affects the sleep-inducing hormone melatonin) for an hour before bedtime.

- Avoid naps later in the day; if you do have one, then keep it under twenty minutes.

- 'Hot bath, cool bedroom' is a good combination for sleep.

- Leave your gadgets in a drawer in the kitchen, turn everything to airplane mode and consider switching off your Wi-Fi at night.

- Clear your mind before you go to bed (try using Robin's simple technique on page 166).

CHAPTER SUMMARY

- Sleep is a key part of the **Health Loop** and is tied in with our circadian rhythm.

- Identifying your chronotype can help you work out what will work best for you in terms of sleep and daily activities.

- Eat dinner early, put your gadgets away, clear your mind and go to bed at the same time every night and wake up each morning at the same time as much as is realistically possible.

8

STRESS

There are not many things you can't physically touch or see that have as huge an effect on us and our health as stress. 'What *is* stress? It's not a real thing, is it?' one of my uncles used to say. He is one of those people who thinks stress is partly what we make it; that it's all in our heads.

But life *is* hard. Grief, illness, loss, that bully at work – all of these can lead to feelings of stress. These are known as 'stressors'.

What causes stress?

Our main stress hormones are cortisol and adrenaline. As I explained on page 94, they serve that fight-or-flight purpose, enabling us to run away from the attacking tiger (or to attempt to fight it), but prolonged stress is, unsurprisingly, bad for us.

In some ways, in simple terms, I think that when we feel extremely stressed – which does happen to all of us at times – it's because our monkey brains have totally hijacked us.

A little bit of stress is good; it helps us perform and gives us enough adrenaline to activate ourselves. But once it tips beyond a certain point, stress leads to a feeling of overwhelm, which is also known as allostatic overload. A study into allostatic load defined allostatic overload as follows:

> *Criterion A: The presence of a current identifiable source of distress in the form of recent life events and/or chronic stress; the stressor is judged to tax or exceed the individual coping skills when its full nature and full circumstances are evaluated.*

> *Criterion B: The stressor is associated with one or more of the following features, which have occurred within six months after the onset of the stressor:*
> 1. *At least two of the following symptoms: difficulty falling asleep, restless sleep, early morning awakening, lack of energy, dizziness, generalised anxiety, irritability, sadness, demoralization*
> 2. *Significant impairment in social or occupational functioning*
> 3. *Significant impairment in environmental mastery (feeling overwhelmed by the demands of everyday life)*[100]

In terms of the sources of your stress, they may be obvious to you, and might leap out at you when you look at your **Health Loop**. If not, you have the tools we have been building throughout this book to help you work them out.

Managing stress

The main ways to manage stress are multipronged.

Firstly, never sweat the small stuff. We have a choice about how to respond to the situations in which we find ourselves. Pay attention to your monkey brain and notice when it is taking over. For example, getting stressed because you are stuck in traffic is pointless, because it's something you cannot do anything about. Also, I think my own stress response to getting stuck in traffic is also partly down to mimicking what I had seen my parents do when I was young. When this happens now, I try to think to myself: 'I genuinely cannot do anything about this... if I'm late, I'm late. At least I'm sure I will get there safely.' This combines two CBT-style exercises we looked at earlier: reframing (see page 104) and adding a positive flip to a negative thought (see page 102).

Secondly, remember to check yourself. The panicky fight-or-flight response is hardwired into us. Our physiology is so clever it knows how to make adrenaline and cortisol send more glucose to the brain and muscles in order to get them ready to 'fight' or run away. While this is great when it helps us swerve out of the way of a careless pedestrian while driving, or catch a falling toddler, if you feel it rear its head inappropriately, there are lots of tools you can deploy.

You could do any of the following for acute stress:

• Stop, take a breath and a moment and THINK before you react.

- Try my one-minute recharge (see page 67) – this can be a great exercise to do if you receive a stressful text, email or letter.

- Drink a glass of water.

- Do some belly breathing (see page 178).

- Try reframing (see page 104).

- Allow yourself to be in the moment and reflect on the situation when you are calmer.

- Remind yourself that you can think rationally by being aware of your monkey brain, which is far more emotional.

Stress prevention

If you have already started some of the practices already mentioned in the book, they should be helping you feel less stressed as time goes on.

Unless you are someone who has a continuous number of serious issues to deal with, day-to-day stress and handling it is about learning to find the sweet spot so that it works for you. The diagram opposite may help you visualise it. It is not always an easy thing to get right, and I do struggle with this myself, but with the right tools and mindset, you can get better at it.

Stress curve

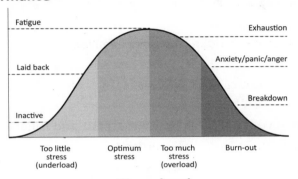

CHAPTER SUMMARY

- Stress is a real thing, and it can affect all of us.

- Recognise that while you may not be able to control a situation, you can control your response to it.

- Learn to notice when your monkey brain is trying to take over with an emotional reaction to a situation.

8

DAILY PREVENTION HACKS

Dental health

Dental issues such as tooth decay, overcrowding and gum disease can lead to other illnesses (including heart disease and respiratory problems), so make an effort to really look after your teeth and gums and have regular check-ups.

The **Deep Dive** on inflammation (see page 116) explains the body's inflammatory response and how it manifests. Bacteria in our gums and teeth can cause an abnormal inflammatory response, potentially leading not just to heart disease, but also Alzheimer's disease and rheumatoid arthritis. The organism *P. gingivalis*, which causes periodontitis (inflammation of the gums), is implicated in these conditions.[101] Getting rid of harmful bacteria and replenishing the population of healthy bacteria in your mouth is the way to go. Rinsing your mouth with salty water can help reduce the amount of harmful bacteria. The mouth has its own flora and the oral microbiome is an interesting area of burgeoning research.[102]

Skin

If you are getting itchy rashes for no reason, but do not have a formal diagnosis like eczema, then:

EXTERNALLY

- Check your products for methylisothiazolinone (MI) or similar. This is a preservative found in shampoos, soaps, sun creams, moisturisers, baby wipes, conditioners and old make-up products. It is a skin sensitiser, so the more you are in contact with it, the more skin irritation it can cause. It can lead to MI allergy.

- Consider softening your water if you can, as this helps to stop the skin from drying out.

- Moisturise straight after a bath or shower without totally drying off, as this locks in the moisture rather than the cream simply skating off the surface of the skin.

- Swap biological soap powders and fabric conditioners for non-bio sensitive skin products.

INTERNALLY

- Stay hydrated with plenty of water.

- Incorporate plenty of omega-3-rich foods in your diet, like walnuts, oily fish and flaxseeds. This may help protect skin against sun damage.

Balance

Walk around barefoot at home. This sounds obvious, but walking barefoot means we have more direct connection with the ground, which can serve to improve our balance via improved proprioception, which is our ability to sense where our joints, muscles and tendons are. The balance exercises on page 185 will help proprioception as well, and should ideally be done barefoot. While mostly essential outdoors, the thick soles of our shoes dampen our proprioceptive abilities.[103]

Water first

Drink a glass of water first thing each morning. This is not for any particular health benefit; it just means that you start your hydration first thing. Poor hydration affects mental performance, skin elasticity and kidney function, and also slows our bowel movements.[104]

Mix things up (a bit)

Although routine is important, for all your habits, variety in *what* you do is key.

Unless you have good reason not to, try to vary what you eat each day in terms of the types of fruits and vegetables you eat, as this will help diversify your gut bacteria.

For exercise, too, variety is good. Think of it as keeping your body guessing. For instance, doing the same aerobic circuits each day sometimes leads to a plateau. Remember the different types of exercise (strength, balance, endurance and flexibility) and rotate them. However, this does not mean doing exercise that does not suit you.

Finally, if all else fails, have self-compassion and 'Act as if...'

If you are struggling with all this behaviour-change work, then there is one simple way to be meta about it. Simply 'act as if'. This does not mean being fake. It means acting as you know you can and would want to.

It's about 'watching' ourselves when we are about to act out using our monkey brains (in other words, when we're about to behave impulsively) and instead doing the opposite.

I have seen this technique at close quarters many times. It's almost like acting like the person you *want* to be in that moment, rather than being led by your monkey brain. In a way, it's a self-check mechanism that can stop you doing things you don't really want to, or might later regret. Think about the roles we fulfil in our lives, both in our jobs and at home. If you can act a certain way in those situations, you can do the same when it comes to benefitting yourself. It is not a perfect method, but is quite a good 'out'.

Most importantly, please do not be hard on yourself.

Make an effort, yes, and by all means learn from mistakes, but none of us are perfect.

Negative self-talk will only make matters worse. Hammering something repeatedly will only stress and weaken it – and that goes for ourselves, too.

8

CONCLUSION: A FEW FINAL WORDS AND THE BEAUTY OF SCIENCE

Now that you have reached the end of this book, I am hoping you have seen that there are logical steps you can take through *The Health Fix* that will improve your health and quality of life. In a world where we question information more than ever, I thought it might be useful to look at how we deduce what really works.

Medicine and healthcare are what they are because of their grounding in science. The scientific method works hard to find the truth. It looks at data, patterns, evidence and best practice.

The difficulty comes when trying to navigate through patchy evidence, or studies with obvious bias (as pointed out in *Bad Pharma* by Professor Ben Goldacre). It is also hard to glean clear direction from areas that are not studied enough, mainly because truly valid studies need funding and the avoidance of bias.

As psychologist Adam Grant says: 'We choose the most convenient arguments to preach our convictions but demand bulletproof facts before we will rethink them.'

This is part of the struggle we have with making recommendations in medicine. What we suggest must do no harm, and what we think works must be based on our take on the best evidence out there.

I remember, many years ago, attending a talk by a professor of public health nutrition who was speaking about added sugars in foods. He was pointing out data that seemed to suggest that low-fat diets were helpful, but I didn't feel there was enough separating out of food items and products in his presentation. I did not agree with him, and asked him about yogurts (which, back then, generally contained both fat and sugar). He said, 'Well, people who eat yogurt are generally very healthy.' It really annoyed me. You cannot on the one hand present data and make statements about the best diet based on certain populations, talking about the 'strength of evidence' and so on, and then bat me down with something woolly and generic about yogurt-eaters being 'generally very healthy' without any hard data there to back it up. Seriously?!

The diagram opposite gives a pictorial definition of evidence-based medicine. Look at the components, and you will see that various factors are combined to reach a decision around treatment. In an ideal world, we would land every consultation in the middle of that Venn diagram, but so often we only manage to hit the overlap of two of the circles.

One of the reasons I want to emphasise individuality is that despite best evidence, and despite good public health messaging, we – as patients and consumers – are all different in our biology and behaviours. Just think of common downstream interventions like medication. Have you ever wondered why ibuprofen works like a dream for you when you sprain your ankle, but makes your sister feel absolutely horrible? Or why one blood pressure tablet works effectively for one person but not at all for another? Pharmaceutical companies have been looking at pharmacogenetics for many years now. This would involve tailoring drugs to our genes and individual receptors (the parts of our cells that receive signals from drugs by which they exert their biological effect).

Part of me is rather impatient and cannot believe we are not already living in that era of medicine, even though there are so many factors to think about before something so specific and costly can be rolled out en masse. My impatience comes from the fact that research and futurism always progress a little more slowly than we might imagine (growing up in the 1970s and 80s, I thought there would be flying cars by '2000 AD'!).

What is evidence-based medicine?

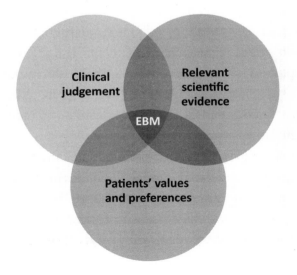

There are certain assumptions that need to be made in order to navigate your health. Medicine is hardly ever a science of exactitude, and of course there are no guarantees.

Basic public health privileges, such as sanitation and access to food, water, light and heat are things all human beings need. I am only too aware that many people on this Earth do not have even those needs met adequately.

But in a way, I wish we lived in a more basic world. The power of 'less' can be wonderful. Years of industrial and technological advances have led to so many so-called advances – like making plastics, processing grains, and the ability to shop and work twenty-four hours a day – that all have an impact on our short- and long-term health and wellbeing.

We have also become obsessed with complexity and specialisation, to the extent that we are moving towards a world where we know more and more about less and less. Add all this to what is happening to the planet in terms of climate change and our oceans, and it is obvious that we need a serious rethink as a society to look at the big picture.

But planetary sustainability aside, *The Health Fix* is all about you and your story. It is different for everyone. It will have given you a way to get your health nearer to where you really want it to be – and, if you want, to keep on improving it.

A lot of people ask me what kind of medicine this is. I don't even know. It is values-based, evolving, progressive, root-cause, behavioural, environmental, 'good' medicine, but it's also partly common sense. Logical and sensible, it was borne out of necessity. I genuinely hope that, like me, you will find this approach life-enriching.

What if nothing happens?

In most cases, this process will help – sometimes a little, sometimes a lot. If you have given it a good shot and feel it is not working, there may be some other established underlying diagnosis that has not yet been detected or some other kind of block or blind spot. Even if you have seen them before, you should probably seek further advice from your healthcare provider.

Good luck – and enjoy the journey

So often in medicine, we learn about disease in order to find out about health. I hope that this book has shown you a way that you can be your own health detective, to monitor, change and ultimately fix problems before they spiral out of control.

Hopefully you will find your **Health Fix** to be a simple and enjoyable process. It starts generically for everyone with the **Health Loop**, but what it ultimately generates is something that is tailored uniquely to you. And you can repeat it as often as you like.

Although focused on you as an individual, I do not want anyone to feel they have to do this on their own. I have already mentioned the power of communities, so I would love for you to share this method with others. Compare notes. Make suggestions to each other. Grow and learn together, as I have with my friends and peers.

When I first started teaching doctors a modified version of this method through my Prescribing Lifestyle Medicine course, I gave them five minutes to do their own **Health Loop** (which was then called the Symptom Web). The amount of chatter in the room and the number of 'aha' moments were staggering.

When I imagine how *The Health Fix* might evolve, I wonder if, in twenty-five years' time, we will be wearing something on our wrists that knows our genetic make-up, and knows which lifestyle interventions and drugs can help us the most as individuals, and can also help us to make the changes we need to, wherever we live in the world.

You now have a toolkit that has the power to improve your health for good. It is a journey that starts with you and finishes with you. As you turn the page to read the final segment of this book, I genuinely hope that it brings welcome changes into your life.

IV

YOUR HEALTH
FIX

"All things are difficult before they are easy."
Thomas Fuller

Now it's your turn to lay things out, make some changes and reflect

Remember that you already have a number of tools and concepts to hand (if you need them) including:

The **IDEAL** framework (for changing behaviours) – page 26

Manage your monkey brain (to control urges) – page 28

Make it fun (to beat the mundane) – page 31

Replacements (to ease yourself out of a bad habit) – page 32

How, What and When? – page 65

Drill Down and Diary Up – page 86

Elimination trial – page 87

Flip exercise (to combat negative thoughts) – page 102

CBT techniques – page 102

Too much vs too little – page 115

Preventing blood glucose spikes – page 132

Core values exercise – page 162

End-of-day ritual – page 166

Smoothie as a shortcut – page 171

Wake up your muscles – page 182

The Daily Prevention Hacks – page 200

and... Remember the power of the **Drawstring Effect**! – page 71
You may or may not need to refer to any of the pages above but feel free to do so if you need a reminder.

Now grab a pen or pencil and get ready to write. If you don't like marking books, then feel free to photocopy the following pages (just don't tell the publisher!). Start by jotting down what your typical day looks like.

YOUR TYPICAL DAY

Morning..
....
....
....
....
....
....
....

Afternoon..
....
....
....
....
....
....
....
....

YOUR TYPICAL DAY

Evening ....

....

....

....

....

....

....

....

Night ....

....

....

....

....

....

....

....

....

Your timeline and medical history

Next, draw out your timeline. Include significant life events and illnesses.

Your Health Loop

Now that you have sketched out your typical day and your time-line, use them to fill out your **Health Loop** which lays out areas which may need some changes.

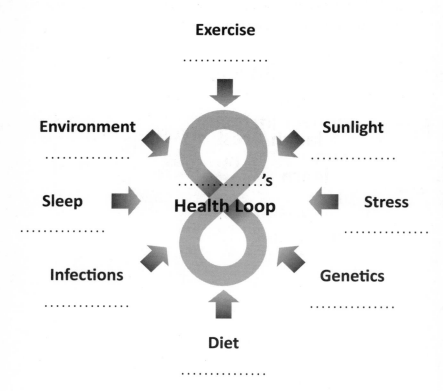

The **Health Loop** will have laid out your story. Now it's time to generate your **Lifestyle Prescription**.

Your Lifestyle Prescription

Take a look at your **Health Loop** and relate it to your typical day. What are the areas that stand out? Is there anything you could change quickly or easily?

Remember, you don't have to do everything in one go. Here are some words that may help you think.

calmer **joy healthier** call
wake breathe kind reading
connect lift compassion nature
laugh rest sleep enjoy slow
sun strong **hug** move run eat
late **learn** savour varied **play** whole
plant love **stretch talk** growing
fun **meditate light water**
supporting walk sing earlier

....

....

....

....

....

....

....
....
....
....
....
....
....
....
....
....
....
....
....
....
....
....
....
....

Weekly reflection

You are likely to notice some changes as you start implementing what you have written out for your **Lifestyle Prescription**. Write down what you have done and what you notice each week.

WEEK 1

....

....

....

....

....

....

....

....

....

....

....

....

WEEK 2

....
....
....
....
....
....
....
....
....
....
....
....
....
....
....
....

WEEK 3

....
....
....
....
....
....
....
....
....
....
....
....
....
....
....
....
....

WEEK 4

....
....
....
....
....
....
....
....
....
....
....
....
....
....
....
....
....

WEEK 5

....
....
....
....
....
....
....
....
....
....
....
....
....
....
....
....
....

WEEK 6

....
....
....
....
....
....
....
....
....
....
....
....
....
....
....
....
....
....

WEEK 7

....

....

....

....

....

....

....

....

....

....

....

....

....

....

....

WEEK 8

....
....
....
....
....
....
....
....
....
....
....
....
....
....
....
....

GENERAL NOTES

....

....

....

....

....

....

....

....

....

....

....

....

....

....

....

....

....

Glossary

ACEs – Adverse Childhood Experiences (traumatic events such as abuse, separation, mental illness or domestic violence).

ADP – adenosine diphosphate, a compound which is important in the role of energy release in cells.

Allele – a version of a gene (we inherit one each for each gene from biological mother and father).

Allostasis – maintaining stability through change (in the context of stress).

Allostatic overload – a state of stress manifesting in various ways including distress, a lack of coping skills, adverse changes to mood, sleep, and significant impairment in functioning.

Alzheimer's disease – the most common type of dementia, a condition in which brain function continues to decline, affecting memory, communication and the ability to perform tasks

Amyloid – a type of protein which can build up in the body's tissues. (Beta-amyloid is specific to Alzheimer's disease).

Anabolic hormone – a hormone such as insulin or growth hormone which stimulates growth and the organisation of molecules.

APOE – a gene which leads to the formation of a protein called Apolipoprotein E.

Apolipoprotein E – a protein which is involved in the transport and metabolism of fats through the bloodstream.

APP – amyloid precursor protein is a molecule that is important for nerve function. It's breakdown can lead to the formation of beta-amyloid in Alzheimer's disease.

ATP – a compound which provides energy to our cells in order for them to carry out various functions.

Autoimmune disease – a disease in which the immune system attacks the body's own tissues and includes rheumatoid arthritis, Hashimoto's Disease, systemic lupus erythematosus, type 1 diabetes, multiple sclerosis and coeliac disease.

Autoimmunity – the process and system by which an individual develops an autoimmune disease (see above).

Automatic behaviours – a behaviour that is usually a result of much repetition and occurs without conscious thinking (such as driving a car).

Bayesian probability-based approach – a method of thinking named after Thomas Bayes' theorem based on data and likelihoods used in situations where there is uncertainty or the answer is not obvious.

Box breathing – a type of breathing involving breathing in for four seconds, then holding the breath for four seconds, breathing out for four seconds and then holding for four seconds before repeating the cycle.

CBT – cognitive behavioural therapy, which is a type of psychological treatment which changes the way one thinks and behaves.

Chromosome – a structure inside the nucleus of our cells made up of DNA, organised into genes. Each of our cells contain twenty-three pairs of chromosomes.

Chronotype – refers to our natural inclination to sleep at a certain time, characterised into morning, evening or neither. They can be characterised into 'animal' subtypes for ease – lion, bear, wolf, and dolphin.

Circadian rhythm – physical, mental and behavioural changes which occur within and follow a twenty-four-hour cycle.

Coeliac disease – an autoimmune condition in which one's immune system attacks the body's tissues in response to eating gluten.

Cortisol – the body's main stress hormone produced in the adrenal glands which are located above the kidneys.

CRP – C-reactive protein, which is a marker of acute inflammation which could be because of infection or another disease state.

Dementia – a progressive condition with varied symptoms affecting the brain, impairing memory, the ability to think, communicate and perform daily activities.

Diary Up – a concept in *The Health Fix* which means looking more carefully at the diary or events leading up to a new or unresolved symptom.

Dopamine – a type of neurotransmitter in the brain primarily involved with pleasure, reward, movement, attention and mood.

Drawstring Effect – coined by myself, specific to *The Health Fix*, describing the phenomenon of 'tightening up'.

Drill Down – for *The Health Fix*, this means eliciting more detailed information about a habit or routine by analysing it.

ECG – electrocardiogram, a tracing of the heart giving some insight into its function.

Epigenetics – how our behaviours and environment can cause changes that affect the way our genes work or are 'expressed'.

Epstein-Barr virus – the virus which causes glandular fever.

ESR – erythrocyte sedimentation rate, a blood marker of inflammation (both acute and longer term).

False belief – something which you think of as 'true' but has no factual basis.

Fibromyalgia – a poorly understood long-term condition which can cause multiple symptoms including pain, fatigue, IBS and brain fog.

Fight-or-flight response – a physiological response of fear or stress preparing us to fight or flee, designed to aid survival in dangerous situations.

Free radicals – reactive, unstable molecules which can cause damage to cells at high concentrations.

GABA – Gamma-aminobutyric acid, a neurotransmitter in the brain which is inhibitory (i.e. slows down nerve transmission).

Genetic marker – a sequence of DNA found on a particular location of a chromosome which can help link an inherited disease with the gene responsible for it.

Glandular fever – often known as the kissing disease, it is a viral condition caused by EBV (Epstein-Barr virus) presenting with fatigue, tonsillitis and sweats.

Glutamate – an excitatory neurotransmitter in the brain.

Gut flora – a synonym for gut microbiota.

H. pylori – *Helicobacter pylori*, a bacterium found in the stomach. Almost half the world are infected with this bacterium but it can cause stomach ulcers and symptoms such as burping or nausea. Certain strains of the bacterium are associated with stomach cancer.

Health Loop – a concept and tool in *The Health Fix* which allows someone to lay out the factors affecting their current state of health.

HLAs – Human leucocyte antigens are a cluster of genes on chromosome 6 that help code proteins which are involved in regulating the immune system and may be linked to autoimmune disease.

Homocysteine – homocysteine is an amino acid in our blood, high levels of which are associated with heart disease, dementia and stroke. It is linked to vitamin B6, vitamin B12 and folate levels in our blood.

Hormone – a hormone is a chemical messenger which is made by a particular organ or gland and then exerts its effect on other parts of the body. Examples include insulin, oestrogen and thyroxine.

How, What and When – literally how, what and when?

IBS – Irritable Bowel Syndrome is a condition which can cause symptoms like stomach cramps, bloating, diarrhoea and constipation.

IDEAL framework – a concept in *The Health Fix* designed to enable behaviour change – Identify, Define, Engage, Activate, Look back.

IgE – Immunoglobulin E, a type of antibody which may indicate allergy.

Inflammogens – anything which causes inflammation in the body.

Intestinal permeability – describes the ability of molecules to cross the lining of the small intestine.

Journalling – writing down your thoughts and feelings.

Lectins – proteins which bind to carbohydrates. Foods containing lectins include beans, nuts and potatoes.

LGG® strain – Lactobacillus GG, also known as *Lactobacillus rhamnosus* is the world's most studied probiotic strain, first isolated by scientists Gorbach and Goldin, hence 'LGG®'.

Lifestyle prescription – recommendations to change habits, environment and behaviours based on your **Health Loop** and typical day.

Long COVID – signs and symptoms that develop during or following an infection consistent with COVID-19 that continue for more than twelve weeks and are not explained by an alternative diagnosis.

Marginal gains – small incremental improvements in a process, such as building habits, which add up to a significant improvement when the increments are added together.

Melatonin – a hormone produced by the pineal gland which helps control our sleep cycle.

Mesolimbic system – part of our central nervous system involving the neurotransmitter dopamine which mediates pleasure and reward.

Methylation – often known as DNA methylation, this is the process of adding a methyl group (one carbon and three hydrogen atoms) to part of our DNA. Methylation changes the way our genes are expressed, thereby potentially changing our risk of developing a disease. This process can be affected by all of the factors in the **Health Loop**.

Methylisothiazolinone (MI) – a chemical which is added to soaps, shampoos, some make-up products as a preservative. It can trigger a skin allergy in the form of contact dermatitis.

Microbiome – a community of microorganisms that live together. The gut microbiome refers to bacteria, viruses, fungi and parasites.

Mitochondria – organelles that generate chemical energy to power a cell's biochemical reactions.

Molecular mimicry – a theoretical term used in biology where a group of peptides (which make up proteins) can be confused by the immune system for another group of peptides because of a similarity in structure. This is how some autoimmune disease is believed to occur.

Monkey brain – our human brains can be considered in three sections – the lizard brain, the monkey brain, and the human brain. The 'lizard' brain is at the base of the brain and is only concerned with our most basic instincts such as fear, fighting, feeding and sleeping. The 'monkey' brain is more expansive and controls emotions. It responds to impulse, wants and desires. The 'human' brain is the 'thinking' part of the brain which is rational and allows us to make considered decisions.

MRI – Magnetic resonance imaging, a type of scanning technology using magnetic fields to produce images of the body.

MTHFR gene – Methylenetetrahydrofolatereductase is an enzyme encoded by the MTHFR gene. It plays a key role in DNA methylation.

NEAT – Non-Exercise Activity Thermogenesis is the energy used to carry out any activity which is not formal exercise.

Non-IgE – a term used to refer to an immune system reaction which does not involve IgE (or Immunoglobulin E) which is one particular type of antibody.

Oxidative stress – a state where there is an excess of free radicals in our cells.

P. gingivalis – a bacterium which can cause periodontitis (gum infection and inflammation) and has been implicated as having a role in the development of coronary heart disease and found in the brain of patients with Alzheimer's disease.

Pacing – a skill involving taking breaks before performing an activity. Pacing allows someone to do as much as they can within their limits.

Periodontitis – often known as periodontal disease, this is infection and inflammation of the gums.

Phyto-oestrogens – oestrogen-like compounds derived from plants such as soybeans and red clover.

Pineal gland – part of our endocrine system and responsible for secreting melatonin.

Prebiotic foods – foods which help increase the amount of beneficial bacteria and fungi in the gut such as garlic, asparagus, onions, leeks, artichokes, bananas, berries and oats.

Probiotic – live microorganisms (usually bacteria but also fungi) which help to restore gut microbiota. Foods like kefir, sauerkraut, kombucha and fermented or pickled foods are probiotic foods. Probiotics are also available in supplement form.

Proprioceptive abilities – the body's ability to perceive its own position in space.

Proton-pump inhibitors – a group of drugs which work on the stomach's proton pumps to stop producing 'excess' acid.

Psoas muscle – large muscle in the lumbar region of the spine which connects the spine to the femur (thigh bone) and is responsible for hip to trunk flexion.

Salivary amylase – an enzyme in saliva which breaks down complex carbohydrates into simple sugars.

Serotonin – an excitatory neurotransmitter in the brain also called 5-HT (5-hydroxytryptamine) involved in the regulation of mood.

SIBO – Small intestinal bacterial overgrowth, a condition which can give rise to symptoms such as bloating after meals, headaches, rashes, joint pains and fatigue.

Systems medicine – a systems-based approach to human biology and medicine appreciating the interconnectedness of our biology.

Tau tangles – 'tangles' of a protein called Tau which can accumulate inside neurons and is a feature of Alzheimer's disease.

Tonsillitis – a viral or bacterial infection of the tonsils.

Toxic positivity – dismissing or ignoring valid negative thoughts or feelings and responding with false reassurance rather than true expression.

Type 2 diabetes – a medical condition whereby blood glucose levels become raised, usually as a result of the body's tissues not being able to respond to one of our hormones, insulin.

Underactive thyroid – known medically as 'hypothyroidism' and confirmed by blood testing, usually accompanied by symptoms which can include tiredness, weight gain, constipation, depression and muscle weakness.

UTI – urinary tract infection.

Vagus nerve – the tenth cranial nerve (arising from the brain) linking the brain to the gastrointestinal tract.

Vascular dementia – a type of dementia caused by disruption of blood flow to the brain.

VDR gene variation – the VDR gene provides instructions for us to respond to vitamin D. Depending on how the proteins in the gene are coded influences how vitamin D is absorbed by an individual.

Endnotes

1   Smith, R. 'Doctors and patients heading in opposite directions'. 1 February 2018. blogs. bmj.com.

2   Tank, A. 'Bill Gates says lazy people make the best employees'. 22 July 2021. entrepreneur. com.

3   Guleria, R., Mathur, V., Dhanuka, A. 'Health Effects of Changing Environment'. *Natural Resource Management: Ecological Perspectives.* 22 March 2019. pp. 95–107.

4   World Health Organization. 'Non-communicable diseases'. 13 April 2021. who.int.

5   Reeve, J., Byng, R. 'Realising the full potential of primary care: uniting the "two faces" of generalism'. *British Journal of General Practice*, vol. 67, no. 660. July 2017. pp.292–3.

6   Professor Tim Spector: www.tim-spector.co.uk

7   Professor Satchidananda Panda: www.salk.edu/scientist/satchidananda-panda

8   Reeve, J., Byng, R. 'Realising the full potential of primary care'.

9   World Health Organization. 'Diarrhoea'. who.int.

10   Husain, M., & Chalder, T. 'Medically unexplained symptoms: assessment and management.' *Clinical medicine (London, England)*, vol. 21, no. 1. 2021. pp 13-18

11   Flores, M., Glusman, G., Brogaard. K., Price, N. D., Hood, L. 'P4 medicine: how systems medicine will transform the healthcare sector and society'. *Personalized Medicine*, vol. 10, no. 6. 2013. pp565–576.

12   Sanvictores, T., Mendez, M. D. 'Types of Parenting Styles and Effects On Children'. StatPearls [Internet]. January 2022.

13   Bernstein, D. M., Coolin, A., Fischer, A. L., Thornton, W. L., Sommerville, J. A. 'False-belief reasoning from 3 to 92 years of age'. PLoS One, vol. 12, no. 9. 29 September 2017.

14   Fogg, B. J. 'Fogg behavior model'. behaviormodel.org

15   Hahn, U. 'The Bayesian boom: good thing or bad?' *Frontiers in Psychology*, vol. 8, no. 5. 8 August 2014. p765.

16   Reeve, J., Byng, R. 'Realising the full potential of primary care'.

17   Yaribeygi, H., Panahi, Y., Sahraei, H., Johnston, T. P., Sahebkar, A. 'The impact of stress on body function: A review'. *EXCLI Journal*, vol. 16. 21 July 2017. pp. 1057–72.

18   National Institute for Health and Care Excellence. 'Tiredness/fatigue in adults: How common is it?'. October 2021. nice.org.uk.

19   Rippe, J. M. 'Lifestyle Medicine: The Health Promoting Power of Daily Habits and Practices'. *American Journal of Lifestyle Medicine*, vol. 12, no. 6. 20 July 2018. pp. 499–512.

20   National Institute for Health and Care Excellence. 'Tiredness/fatigue in adults'. https://cks.nice.org.uk/topics/tiredness-fatigue-in-adults/background-information/ prevalence/

21   Willacy, H. 'Fatigue and TATT'. 30 April 2019. patient.info.

22   Yaribeygi, H. *et al.* 'The impact of stress on body function'.

23   Elvers, K. T, Wilson, V. J., Hammond, A., et al. 'Antibiotic-induced changes in the human gut microbiota for the most commonly prescribed antibiotics in primary care in the UK: a systematic review'. *BMJ Open.* 21 September 2020.

24   Fields, H. 'The Gut: Where bacteria and immune system meet'. November 2015. hopkinsmedicine.org.

25   Madison, A., Kiecolt-Glaser, J. K. 'Stress, depression, diet, and the gut microbiota: human-bacteria interactions at the core of psychoneuroimmunology and nutrition'. *Current Opinion in Behavioral Sciences*, vol. 28. August 2019. pp.105–110.

26   DiBaise, M., Tarleton, S. M. 'Hair, Nails, and Skin: Differentiating Cutaneous Manifestations of Micronutrient Deficiency'. *Nutrition in Clinical Practice*, vol. 34, no. 4. Aug 2019. pp. 490–503.

27   Aguayo-Patrón, S. V., Calderón de la Barca, A.M. 'Old Fashioned vs. Ultra-Processed-Based Current Diets: Possible Implication in the Increased Susceptibility to Type 1 Diabetes and Celiac Disease in Childhood'. *Foods*, vol. 6, no. 11. 15 November 2017.

28   Gerritsen, R. J. S., Band, G. P. H. 'Breath of Life: The Respiratory Vagal Stimulation Model of Contemplative Activity'. *Frontiers in Human Neuroscience*, vol. 12. 9 October 2018. p. 397.

29   Carlson, J. L., Erickson, J. M., Lloyd, B. B., Slavin, J. L. 'Health Effects and Sources of Prebiotic Dietary Fiber'. *Current Developments in Nutrition*, vol. 2, no. 3. 29 January 2018.

30   Segers, M. E., Lebeer, S. 'Towards a better understanding of *Lactobacillus rhamnosus GG*--host interactions'. *Microbial Cell Factories*, vol. 13. 29 August 2014.

31   Cecilio, L. A., Bonatto, M. W. 'The prevalence of HLA DQ2 and DQ8 in patients with celiac disease, in family and in general population'. *Arquivos Brasileiros de Cirurgia Digestiva*, vol. 28, no. 3. July–September 2015. pp. 183–5.

32   Moore, J. G., Datz, F. L., Christian, P. E., Greenberg, E., Alazraki, N. 'Effect of body posture on radionuclide measurements of gastric emptying'. *Digestive Diseases and Sciences*, vol. 33, no. 12. December 1988. pp. 1592–5.

33   El Menabawey, T., Dluzewski, S., Phillpotts, S., *et al.* 'PTU-112 Proton Pump Inhibitors – A Risk for Micronutrient Deficiency. But Are We Looking Out for This?' *Gut*, vol. 65. 2016.

34   Rao, S. S. C., Bhagatwala, J. 'Small Intestinal Bacterial Overgrowth: Clinical Features and Therapeutic Management'. *Clinical and Translational Gastroenterology*, vol. 10, no. 10. October 2019.

35   Camilleri, M. 'Leaky gut: mechanisms, measurement and clinical implications in humans'. *Gut*, vol. 68, no. 8. August 2019. pp. 1516–26

36   Paray, B. A., Albeshr, M. F., Jan, A. T., Rather, I. A. 'Leaky Gut and Autoimmunity: An Intricate Balance in Individuals Health and the Diseased State'. *International Journal of Molecular Sciences*, vol. 21, no. 24. 21 December 2020. p. 9770

37   Firoze Khan, M., Wang, H. 'Autoimmune diseases: Contribution of gut microbiome'. *Frontiers in Immunology*. 10 January 2020. frontiersin.org.

38   National Institute for Health and Care Excellence. 'Vitamin D: supplement use in specific population groups'. 30 August 2017. nice.org.uk.

39   Jo. J., Garssen, J., Knippels. L., Sandalova, E. 'Role of cellular immunity in cow's milk allergy: pathogenesis, tolerance induction, and beyond'. *Mediators of Inflammation*. 9 June 2014.

40   Cusick, M .F., Libbey, J. E., Fujinami, R. S. 'Molecular mimicry as a mechanism of autoimmune disease'. *Clinical Reviews in Allergy and Immunology*, vol. 42, no. 1. February 2012. pp. 102–11.

41   Mastrorilli, C., Cardinale, F., Giannetti, A., & Caffarelli, C. 'Pollen-Food Allergy Syndrome: A not so Rare Disease in Childhood'. *Medicina (Kaunas, Lithuania)*, vol. 55, no 10. October 2019. pp 641

42   Gong, T., Wang, X., Yang, Y., Yan, Y., Yu, C., Zhou, R., Jiang, W. 'Plant Lectins Activate the NLRP3 Inflammasome To Promote Inflammatory Disorders'. *Journal of Immunology*, vol. 198, no 5. 1 March 2017. pp. 2082–92

43   World Health Organization. 'Depression'. who.int.

44   Holland, K. 'Everything you need to know about anxiety'. 28 June 2022. healthline.com

45   World Health Organization. 'Mental Health'. who.int.

46   World Health Organization. 'Mental Health: Strengthening our Response'. 17 June 2022. who.int.

47   A. H. Maslow (1943). Originally Published in 'Psychological Review', 50, 370-396.

48   Chang, X., Jiang, X., Mkandarwire, T., Shen, M. 'Associations between adverse childhood experiences and health outcomes in adults aged 18–59 years'. *PLoS One*, vol. 14, no. 2. 7 February 2019.

49   National Health Service. 'An introduction to the NHS'. nhs.uk.

50   . Werner. 'The children of Kauai: Resiliency and recovery in adolescence and adulthood'. *Journal of Adolescent Health*. vol 13, no. 4. 1992. Pp. 262-268.

51   Institute for Quality and Efficiency in Health Care (IQWiG). 'Cognitive behavioural therapy'. 7 August 2013. informedhealth.org.

52   Keown, P., Mercer, G., Scott, J. 'Retrospective analysis of hospital episode statistics, involuntary admissions under the Mental Health Act 1983, and number of psychiatric beds in England 1996-2006'. *British Medical Journal*. 2008. p. 337

53   Shadrina, M., Bondareno, E. A., Slominksy, P. A. 'Genetics factors in major depression disease'. *Frontiers in Psychiatry*. 23 July 2018. frontiersin.org.

54   Mattar, R., de Campos Mazo, D. F., Carrilho, F. J. 'Lactose intolerance: diagnosis, genetic, and clinical factors'. *Clinical and Experimental Gastroenterology*, vol 5. 2012. pp. 113–21.

55   Casaubon, J. T., Kashyap, S. Regan, J. P. 'BRCA1 and 2'. StatPearls [Internet]. 22 September 2021.

56   Nyholt, D. R., Yu, C. E., Visscher, P. M. 'On Jim Watson's APOE status: genetic information is hard to hide'. *European Journal of Human Genetics*, vol. 17, no. 2. February 2009. pp. 147–9.

57   Turgal, M., Gumruk, F., Karaagaoglu, E., Beksac, M. S. 'Methylenetetrahydrofolate Reductase Polymorphisms and Pregnancy Outcome'. *Geburtshilfe Frauenheilkd*, vol. 78, no. 9. September 2018. pp. 871–8.

58   Liguori, I., Russo, G., Curcio, F., Bulli, G., Aran, L., Della-Morte, D., Gargiulo, G., Testa, G., Cacciatore, F., Bonaduce, D., Abete, P. 'Oxidative stress, aging, and diseases'. *Clinical Interventions in Aging*, vol. 13. 26 April 2018. pp.757–72.

59   Liguori *et al.* 'Oxidative stress, aging and diseases'.

60   Rudrapal, M., Khairnar, S. J., Khan, J., Dukhyil, A. B., Ansari, M. A., Alomary, M. N., Alshabrmi, F. M., Palai, S, Deb Prashanta, K., Devi, R. 'Dietary Polyphenols and Their Role in Oxidative Stress-Induced Human Diseases: Insights Into Protective Effects, Antioxidant Potentials and Mechanism(s) of Action'. *Frontiers in Pharmacology*, vol 13. 2022.

61   Alzheimer's Research UK. 'Global prevalance'. Dementia Statistics Hub. dementiastatistics.org.

62   Gómez-Pinilla, F. 'Brain foods: the effects of nutrients on brain function'. *Nature Reviews Neurosciences*, vol. 9, no. 7. pp. 568–78.

63   Zilliox, L. A., Chadrasekaran, K., Kwan, J. Y., Russell, J. W. 'Diabetes and Cognitive Impairment'. *Current Diabetes Reports*, vol. 16, no. 9. September 2016. p. 87.

64   Zárate, S., Stevnsner, T., Gredilla, R. 'Role of Estrogen and Other Sex Hormones in Brain Aging. Neuroprotection and DNA Repair'. *Frontiers in Aging Neuroscience*, vol. 9. 22 December 2017. p. 430.

65   World Health Organization. 'Global Dementia Observatory'. who.int.

66   Edwards III, G. A., Gamez, N., Escobedo, G. Jr, Calderon, O., Moreno-Gonzalez, I. 'Modifiable Risk Factors for Alzheimer's Disease'. *Frontiers in Aging Neuroscience*, vol. 11. 24 June 2019. p. 146.

67   Taylor, R. 'Insulin resistance and type 2 diabetes'. *Diabetes*, vol. 61, no. 4. April 2012. pp. 778–9.

68   Facchini, F. S., Hua, N., Abbasi, F., Reaven, G. M. 'Insulin resistance as a predictor of age-related diseases'. *Journal of Clinical Endocrinology and Metabolism*, vol. 86, no. 6. August 2001. pp. 3574–8.

69   Mohammady, M., Janani, L., Jahanfar, S., Mousavi, M. S. 'Effect of omega-3 supplements on vasomotor symptoms in menopausal women: A systematic review and meta-analysis'. *European Journal of Obstetrics & Gynecology and Reproductive Biology*. September 2018. pp. 295–302.

70   The Hoffman Institute. 'Trauma, resilience and addiction: Hoffman interviews Dr Gabor Maté'. hoffmaninstitute.co.uk

71   Yanguas, J., Pinazo-Henandis, S., Tarazona-Santabalbina, F. J. 'The complexity of loneliness'. *Acta Biomedica*, vol. 89, no. 2. 7 June 2018. pp. 302–314.

72   Raveendran, A. V., Jayadevan, R., Sashidharan, S. 'Long COVID: An overview'. *Diabetology & Metabolic Syndrome*, vol. 15, no. 3. May–June 2021. pp. 869–75.

73   Shikova, E., Reshkova, V., Kumanova, A., Raleva, S., Alexandrova, D., Capo, N., Murovska, M. European Network on ME/CFS (EUROMENE). 'Cytomegalovirus, Epstein-Barr virus, and human herpesvirus-6 infections in patients with myalgic encephalomyelitis/ chronic fatigue syndrome'. *Journal of Medical Virology*, vol. 92, no. 12. 4 March 2020. pp. 3682–8.

74   Martínez-Lara, A., Moreno-Fernández, A. M., Jiménez-Guerrero, M., Díaz-López, C., De-Miguel, M., Cotán, D., Sánchez-Alcázar, J. A. 'Mitochondrial Imbalance as a New Approach to the Study of Fibromyalgia'. *Open Access Rheumatology*, vol. 12. 24 August 2020. pp. 175–85.

75   Hernández-Camacho, J. D., Bernier, M., López-Lluch, G., Navas, P. 'Coenzyme Q10 Supplementation in Aging and Disease'. *Frontiers in Physiology*, vol. 9. 5 February 2018. p. 44.

76   Stohs, S. J., Chen, O., Ray, S. D., Ji, J., Bucci, L. R., Preuss, H. G. 'Highly Bioavailable Forms of Curcumin and Promising Avenues for Curcumin-Based Research and Application: A Review'. *Molecules*, vol 25, no. 6. 19 March 2020. p. 1397.

77   Nagpal, M., Sood, S. 'Role of curcumin in systemic and oral health: An overview'. *Journal of Natural Science, Biology and Medicine*, vol. 4, no. 1. January 2013. pp. 3–7.

78   Markowiak, P., Ślieżewska, K. 'Effects of Probiotics, Prebiotics, and Synbiotics on Human Health'. *Nutrients*, vol 9, no. 9. 15 September 2017. p. 1021.

79   Carrasco-Gallardo, C., Guzmán, L., Maccioni, R. B. 'Shilajit: a natural phytocomplex with potential procognitive activity'. *International Journal of Alzheimer's Disease*. 2012.

80   Li, Y., Yao, J., Han, C., Yang, J., Chaudhry, M. T., Wang, S., Liu, H., Yin, Y. 'Quercetin, Inflammation and Immunity'. *Nutrients*, vol. 8, no. 3. 15 March 2016. p. 167.

81   Reimers, A., Ljung, H. 'The emerging role of omega-3 fatty acids as a therapeutic option in neuropsychiatric disorders'. *Therapeutic Advances in Psychopharmacology*, vol. 9. 24 June 2019.

82   Swanson, D., Block, R., Mousa, S. A. 'Omega-3 fatty acids EPA and DHA: health benefits throughout life'. *Advances in Nutrition*, vol. 3, no. 1. January 2012. pp. 1–7.

83   Yubero-Serrano, E. M., Lopez-Moreno, J., Gomez-Delgado, F., Lopez-Miranda, J. 'Extra virgin olive oil: More than a healthy fat'. *European Journal of Clinical Nutrition*, vol. 72. July 2019. pp. 8–17.

84   Mollazadeh, H., Hosseinzadeh, H. 'Cinnamon effects on metabolic syndrome: a review based on its mechanisms'. *Iranian Journal of Basic Medical Sciences*, vol. 19, no. 12. December 2016. pp. 1258–70.

85   Nagpal and Sood. 'Role of curcumin in systemic and oral health'.

86   Ansary, J., Forbes-Hernández, T. Y., Gil, E., Cianciosi, D., Zhang, J., Elexpuru-Zabaleta, M., Simal-Gandara, J., Giampieri, F., Battino, M. 'Potential Health Benefit of Garlic Based on Human Intervention Studies: A Brief Overview'. *Antioxidants*, vol. 9, no. 7. 15 July 2020. p. 619.

87   Isbill, J., Kandiah, J., Kružliaková, N. 'Opportunities for Health Promotion: Highlighting Herbs and Spices to Improve Immune Support and Well-being'. *Integrative Medicine*, vol 19, no. 5. October 2020. pp. 30–42.

88 Isbill, J., *et al.* 'Opportunities for Health Promotion'.

89 Isbill, J., *et al.* 'Opportunities for Health Promotion'.

90 Isbill, J., et al. 'Opportunities for Health Promotion'.

91 LIczbiński, P., & Bukowska, B. 'Tea and coffee polyphenols and their biological properties based on the latest *in vitro* investigations'. *Industrial crops and products*, vol. 175. 2022.

92 Koga. K., Taguchi, A., Koshimizu, S., Suwa, Y., Yamada, Y., Shirasaka, N., Yoshizumi, H. 'Reactive oxygen scavenging activity of matured whiskey and its active polyphenols'. *Journal of Food Science*, vol. 72, no. 3. April 2007. pp.S212–7.

93 Finch, L. E. , Tomiyama, A. J., Ward, A. 'Taking a Stand: The Effects of Standing Desks on Task Performance and Engagement'. *International Journal of Environmental Research and Public Health*, vol. 14, no. 8. 21 August 2017. p. 939.

94 Ardeljan AD, Hurezeanu R. Sarcopenia. [Updated 2022 Jul 4]. In: StatPearls [Internet]. Treasure Island (FL): StatPearls Publishing; 2022 Jan.

95 Chung, N., Park, M. Y., Kim, J., Park, H. Y., Hwang, H., Lee, C. H., Han, J. S., So, J., Park, J., Lim K. 'Non-exercise activity thermogenesis (NEAT): a component of total daily energy expenditure'. *Journal of Exercise Nutrition & Biochemistry*, vol. 22, no. 2. 30 June 2018. pp. 23–30.

96 Bennett, W. C., & Zingg, R. M. 'The Tarahumara: an Indian tribe of northern Mexico'. 1935.

97 Chung, N. *et al.* 'Non-exercise activity thermogenesis (NEAT)'.

98 Worley, S. L. 'The Extraordinary Importance of Sleep: The Detrimental Effects of Inadequate Sleep on Health and Public Safety Drive an Explosion of Sleep Research'. *Physical Therapy*, vol. 43, no. 12. December 2018. pp. 758–63.

99 Montaruli, A., Castelli, L., Mulè, A., Scurati, R., Esposito, F., Galasso, L., Roveda, E. 'Biological Rhythm and Chronotype: New Perspectives in Health'. *Biomolecules*, vol 11, no. 4. 24 March 2021. p. 487.

100 Guidi, J., Lucente, M., Sonino, N., Fava, G. A. 'Allostatic Load and Its Impact on Health: A Systematic Review'. *Psychotherapy and Psychosomatics*, vol. 90, no. 1. 2021. pp. 11–27.

101 Sanz, M., del Castillo, A. M., Jepsen, S., Gonzalez-Juanatey, J. R., D'Aiuto, F., et al. 'Periodontitis and cardiovascular diseases: Consensus report'. *Journal of Clinical Periodontology*, vol. 47, no. 3. 3 February 2020. pp. 268–88.

102 Campbell, K. 'Oral microbiome findings challenge dentistry dogma'. 27 October 2021. nature.com.

103 Franklin, S., Li, F. X., Grey, M. J. 'Modifications in lower leg muscle activation when walking barefoot or in minimalist shoes across different age-groups'. *Gait & Posture*, vol. 60. February 2018. pp. 1–5.

104 Armstrong, L. E., Johnson, E. C. 'Water Intake, Water Balance, and the Elusive Daily Water Requirement'. *Nutrients*, vol. 10, no. 12. 5 December 2018. p. 1928.

Index

ability, and behaviour change
      21–2, 25
acceptance 167
ACEs (adverse childhood
      experiences) 97–8
      aches and pains 83–92
      experiences of pain 83–4
      Health Loop for 84, 85–6, 88, 92
      Raphael's typical day 85, 86
'act as if' 203–4
activating, in the IDEAL framework
      26, 27–9
acute medicine 110
ADHD 105
ADP molecule 149
adrenaline 195, 199
alcohol 128, 142, 173, 193
allergy and inflammation 90–1
allostatic overload 195–6
Alzheimer's disease 48, 105, 107,
      108, 117, 120, 122, 125–9, 133, 190
      and genetics 125–8
anaemia 57
antibiotics 62, 63, 78, 115
antioxidants 135
anxiety 93, 166
APOE gene 125–6
APP (amyloid precursor protein)
      127–8
arthritis 88
ATP molecule 149
autoimmune diseases 70–1, 79–81,
      84
      coeliac disease 57, 59
autonomic nervous system 153

back pain 183
balance exercises 185, 202
Baldwin, James 155
barefoot walking 202
Baysian probability approach 37
BDNF (brain-derived neurotrophic
      factor) 48, 151
behavioural change 19–21, 25, 53,
      159–60
      'act as if' 203–4
      and exercise 189
      IDEAL framework for 26–34,
            35, 52, 112, 121, 130, 136, 143,
            158, 163
      reasons for 22–5
      systems and symptoms 40–2, 56
behavioural processes 18–25
      behavioural theory 21–2
      being defined by 19–20
      see also monkey brain
belly breathing 67, 109, 166, 178–9,
      180, 198
beta-amyloid 127–8
bias in scientific studies 205
biological processes 18
biological systems 46–8
      and symptoms 36–40
birch pollen allergy 91
bloating 64, 79
blood glucose 173, 174
      and insulin levels 131–4
blood platelets 151
blood pressure
      checking 58
      tiredness and fatigue 62

blood sugar levels 131, 134
blood tests 58, 59, 61, 77, 84, 98, 111, 124
boring tasks, making fun 31–2
brain
    and Alzheimer's 127–8
    BDNF (brain-derived neurotrophic factor) 48, 151
    and behaviour 18
    and dopamine 131
    and memory problems 121, 122–3
    and the nervous system 38, 39, 41, 47, 124
    scans 123
breast cancer 107
breathing exercises 109, 176, 178–9
    belly breathing 67, 109, 166, 178–9, 180, 198
    for tiredness and fatigue 60, 67

caffeine 173, 193
cancer 117, 134
carbon monoxide poisoning 115, 119
cardiovascular system 38, 39, 41, 47, 133
carpal tunnel syndrome 183
case studies 56
    Amelia (tiredness and fatigue) 57–73, 79, 81
    Gary (digestive problems) 74–82
    Janine (memory problems) 121–4, 129–37
    Johnny (feelings of illness) 138–44

Martha (Covid recovery) 145–54
Norah (mystery illness) 11–16, 119
Raphael (aches and pains) 83–92
Shane (mental health) 95–105
CBT (cognitive behaviour therapy) 102–4, 109, 197
childhood experiences, influence on behaviour 19
chronic fatigue 151
chronic pain 45
circadian rhythm 190–1, 192
co-enzyme Q10 (antioxidant) 150–1
coeliac disease 57, 59, 62, 69–71, 105
coffee 135, 173
cognitive behaviour therapy (CBT) 102–4, 109, 197
community spirit, and behaviour change 24, 25
concentration, tiredness and fatigue 62
cortisol 62, 195, 197
Couch to 5K 130
COVID recovery 12, 56, 145–52
    energy and post-viral fatigue 149
    exercise 148–9
    medication 148
    symptoms 145
curcumin 129

da Vinci, Leonardo 17
deep dives 15, 56
    allergy and inflammation 90–1
    Alzheimer's 125–9
    chronic inflammation 116–19

coeliac disease 69–71
genes and mental health 104–8
the gut and autoimmunity 79–81
and memory problems 136
dementia 120–1
see also Alzheimer's disease
dental health 200
depression 93, 94, 105–7
antidepressant medication 98
desk-based workers, and exercise
176–7
diabetes 125, 176
pre-diabetic 124
type 1 81
type 2 48, 85, 128, 131, 132, 190
diarrhoea 64, 70
diary up 15
aches and pains 87–8, 89, 92
mystery illnesses 113–15
diet see food and diet
digestive problems 74–82
drawstring effects 79
Health Loop 75–8
dopamine 33, 131
drawstring effect 15, 138, 143
digestive problems 79
mental health 100
post-viral recovery 152
tiredness and fatigue 71–2, 73
drill down 15
aches and pains 86–7, 89, 92
mystery illnesses 113–15

ear infections 75, 77–8
endocrine system (hormones) 38,
39, 41, 47, 48, 124
energy, tiredness and fatigue 62
engaging, in the IDEAL framework
26, 30–1

environment change 30–1
epigenetics 127
Epstein-Barr virus 58, 147
evidence-based medicine 205
exercise 117, 176–89
balance 185, 202
benefits of 47–8
and COVID recovery 148–9
desk-based workers 176–7
in the Health Loop 44, 45
invisible 'exercise' 186
and memory problems 129–30
movement 176–7, 179–82
running 185, 186
and sleep 193
variety in 202–3
wake-up routine 165–6, 180–2
walking 184, 185, 187
external rules and restrictions, and
behaviour change 23
extra-virgin olive oil 171

fatty liver disease 133
fibromyalgia 84, 149
Fixes 14–15
flight-or-fight response 94–5, 195,
197
Fogg, Professor B.J. 21, 25, 27
food and diet 168–75
ad hoc cooking 32
anti-inflammatory diet 149
antioxidant-rich foods 117
breakfast 174
coffee 135, 173
and the drawstring effect 71–2
eating while standing 76, 77
eliminating foods 92, 171
extra-virgin olive oil 171

fast/junk food 30, 31, 32–3
food diaries 92
herbs and spices 171–3
high-fibre foods 169
and the immune system 73
lectins 88–9
and memory problems 122,
    130–3, 136
and mental health 100, 101
milk allergies 90–1
mindful eating 168
nutrient-rich foods 170–1
omega-3 rich foods 201
and the peri-menopause 135–6
probiotics 68, 69
processed food 66–7, 128, 172
    refined carbs 131
reducing food waste 32
smoothies 169
sugary foods 33–4, 130–2
time-related eating 131, 132–3,
    134, 137, 174, 193
and tiredness and fatigue 59,
    60, 61, 64, 66–7, 68
variety in 202
whole foods 66, 68, 78, 128, 169
Foster, Jeff 7
free radicals 116, 117, 135, 171
Fuller, Thomas 211

gastrointestinal system 38, 39, 41, 47
    and memory problems 124
Gates, Bill 9
genetic testing 107–8
genetics
    Alzheimer's 125–8
    and autoimmunity 81
    coeliac disease 69–71

in the Health Loop 44, 45, 58
and mental health 104–8, 109
NDR gene variation 164
tiredness and fatigue 62
glandular fever 58, 146–7
gout 88
Grant, Adam 205
gut bacteria/flora 68, 79, 151, 173
    and antibiotics 63–4, 78
    and autoimmunity 79–81

habits
activating 27–8
bad habits and managing your
    monkey brain 28–9
and behaviour 20–1
and the drawstring effect 72
happy accidents, and behaviour
    change 23
harmful habits 20–1
health coaching 98
Health Fix toolkit 52–3, 106, 163–4
'health is wealth' 9, 56
Health Loop 15, 42–6, 50, 52, 53, 56,
    158, 209, 210, 216–17
    aches and pains 84, 85–6, 88, 92
    Alzheimer's 125, 128
    and the brain 121, 123, 124
    diet 44, 45
    digestive problems 75–8
    and the drawstring effect 71
    environment 44, 46
    exercise 44, 45
    feelings of illness 139, 143, 144
    genetics 44, 45, 58
    infections 44, 45–6
    interconnectedness of 163, 164
    long COVID 147

memory problems 129
mental health 97, 100, 104–5, 106
mystery illness 111, 112–13
sleep 44, 46, 190, 193
and stress 44, 45, 196
    one-minute recharge 67–8,
        101, 109
    sunlight 44, 45
    tiredness and fatigue 60–2, 63,
        65–9
heart disease 105, 108, 117, 190
heartburn 74–5, 78
herbs 171–3
HHV6 virus 151
high blood pressure 57
HLAs, and coeliac disease 69–71
homocysteine 108
hormones (endocrine system) 38,
    39, 41, 47, 48, 124
How, What and When questions
    15, 66
    Alzheimer's 128
    diet 168–9
    digestive problems 76–7
    memory problems 131
HRT (hormone replacement
    therapy) 135

IBS (irritable bowel syndrome) 79
IDEAL framework for behavioural
    change 26–34, 35, 52, 112, 121,
    143, 158, 163
    and memory problems 130, 136
illness, feelings of 138–44
immune system 38, 39, 41, 173
    coeliac disease 69–70
    dysfunction 117, 118
    gut bacteria 68

and memory problems 124
    and molecular mimicry 90–1
    and processed food 67
    tiredness and fatigue 62, 63–4
individuality 206–7, 209
infections, in the Health Loop 44,
    45–6
inflammation 116–19, 151, 171
    and allergy 90–1
    and dental health 200
insulin resistance 48, 131, 132, 135,
    137
interconnected systems 48
iron deficiency 65, 66

lectins 88–9
lifestyle 95
    defining 49
Lifestyle Prescriptions 15, 48–9, 50,
    52, 53, 56, 158, 163, 210, 219
    COVID recovery 149, 153
    feelings of illness 144
    memory problems 124, 129–35
    mental health 101
    tiredness and fatigue 59, 66–9, 71
lupus 88
Lyme disease 58

marginal gains, power of 28, 78,
    172, 189
medical history 49, 50
medically unexplained symptoms 13
medicine, symptoms in 36–8
meditation 149–50, 159
melatonin 192, 193
memory problems 120–37
    blood glucose and insulin levels
        131–4

and the brain 121, 122–3
and exercise 129–30
food and diet 122, 130–3, 136
and lifestyle tweaks 135–6
menopause 106
peri-menopause 124, 135–6
mental health 93–109
ACEs (adverse childhood
experiences) 97–8
and CBT (cognitive behaviour
therapy) 102–4, 109
depression 93, 94, 105–7
and genes 104–8, 109
Health Loop 97, 100, 104–5, 106
resilience 99–100
methylation 108
microbiome 64, 79, 89, 151
oral 200
micronutrient deficiency 65
milk allergies 90–1
miscarriage 107–8
mitochandria 149
mitochondria 184
molecular mimicry 90–1
monkey brain 35, 52, 103
and 'act as if' 203–4
awareness of 159, 163
and bad habits 28–9
and replacements 32–4
and stress 195, 197, 198
and the trauma-pain-addiction
cycle 143–4
motivation, and behaviour change
21–2, 25
movement 176–7, 179–82
MTHFR gene 108
musculoskeletal system 38, 39,
41, 124

mystery symptoms 110–19

NEAT (non-exercise activity
thermogenesis) 186
negative thoughts, flip exercise for
101–2, 197
nervous system (brain) 38, 39, 41,
47, 124
nuanced self-analysis, and
memory problems 136–7
nutrient-rich foods 170–1

oestrogen 124, 136
omega-3 fatty acids 136, 151–2, 201
one-minute recharge 67–8, 101,
109, 166, 198
oxidative stress 116, 118

pacing 148–9
pain see aches and pains
Panda, Satchidenada 11
Peile, Ed 156
pharmacogenetics 207
pigeon pose 182
polycystic ovarian syndrome 134
polymorphisms 105
polyphenols 135
post-viral syndrome 146–7
posture 177
prayer 159
and post-viral recovery 148,
149–50
probiotic supplements 78, 81, 151
probiotics 68, 69
processed food 66–7, 128, 172
refined carbohydrates 131
prompts, and behaviour change
21–2, 25

prostatitis 115
proton-pump inhibitors 77
psoas muscle 181

quercetin 151

reading 159
relaxation, and the drawstring
    effect 72
replacements 32–4
reproductive system 124
resilience 99–100
resolution 166
rules and restrictions, and
    behaviour change 23
running 185, 186

sacopenia 177
Saving Lives in Slow Motion
    (podcast) 6
Seneca 55
shilajit 151
SIBO (small intestinal bacterial
    overgrowth) 79–81
skin rashes 201
sleep 10, 117, 190–4, 196
    and Alzheimer's 128
    chronotypes 190–2
    end-of-day ritual 166, 194
    in the Health Loop 44, 46, 190, 193
    naps 193
    poor sleep 32, 52, 190
        tiredness and fatigue 60, 61
    tips for 192–4
    tiredness and fatigue 62
smartphones
    addiction-withdrawal
        behaviour 33

    days of doing without 30–1
smoking 128, 142, 157–8
smoothies 169
social media, and the monkey
    brain 33
Spector, Tim 11
spices 171–3
stress 195–9
    and Alzheimer's 128
    causes of 195–6
    and digestive problems 77
    flight-or-fight response 94–5,
        195, 197
    in the Health Loop 44, 45, 196
    management 197–8
    one-minute recharge 67–8, 101,
        109, 166, 198
    prevention 198–9
    and tiredness and fatigue
        (Amelia) 61–2, 67
stressful events, tiredness and
    fatigue 59, 61
strokes 121, 157
sugary foods 33–4, 130–2
suicide 93
sunlight, in the Health Loop 44, 45
supplements 148, 150–3, 154
    probiotic 68, 69, 151
    vitamins 152–3
Symptom Web 43
symptoms
    and biological systems 36–40
    Health Loop 42–6
    and lifestyle 49
    and systems 36–53, 40–2, 65,
        79, 94
systems malfunction 117
    water leak analogy 42–3, 46

systems medicine 38–40

Tarahumaras peoples 185, 186
TATT (tired all the time) 57
tea 173
thyroid, underactive 57
timelines 63, 139–42, 215
tiredness and fatigue 57–73
    drawstring effect 71–2, 73
    food and diet 59, 60, 61, 64,
       66–7, 68
    Health Loop 60–2, 63, 65–9
    medical reasons for 57
    TATT (tired all the time) 57
trauma-pain-addiction cycle
    143–4
trigger events, and behaviour
    change 24, 25
turmeric 151
type 2 diabetes 48, 57, 85, 128, 131,
    132, 190
typical days 49, 213–14, 217

unpredictable events 158–9
urine infections 59, 61

vagus nerve 67, 68, 150, 179
values, identifying core values
    160–2
vascular dementia 120–1
vitamins
    deficiencies
        B vitamins 57, 59, 77, 124, 125
        vitamin D 57, 59, 77, 105, 125,
           164
    supplements 152–3
    vitamin D 57, 59, 61, 85, 129

wake-up routine 165–6, 180–2
walking 184, 185, 187
washing-up 31–2
water intake 68, 169, 173, 174
Watson, James 107
Werner, Dr Emmy 99
whole foods 66, 68, 78, 128, 169
willpower, and behaviour change
    18, 25

Acknowledgements

I won't lie. **The Health Fix** has been a difficult labour of love written in snatched moments after brutally long days at work. Nights, weekends, annual leave were all-consuming and all interspersed with a family wedding and two family funerals. There was no long sabbatical by a lake, no ghostwriting buddy or any kind of creative retreat. But we got there.

As I was writing, I held firm in my mind patients, their experiences and the skill of some wonderful teachers and healthcare practitioners I have learnt from and worked with over the last thirty years, both in and outside of the NHS. It is because of you that my purpose for this book is so strong and the reason I managed to complete it.

None of this would have happened without the team at Kyle – my truly steadfast publisher Joanna Copestick who believed in the book, editor Samhita Foria with an eagle eye for detail and overkill, and copy editor Tara O'Sullivan who has spared me a blush or two. And without Megan Brown, Rosa Patel, Melissa Baker, Alice Groser, Liam Wheatley, Paul Palmer-Edwards, Lucy Carter, Nic Jones and Mel Four, this book would not stir the senses as much as I hope it does.

Jon Fowler – thank you for championing me my friend.

The list of friends I need to thank is long. You have helped shape this book more than you know – Rangan Chatterjee, Jeremy Hawkey, Rupy Aujla, Gemma Newman, Sunetra Sarker, the Kent weekender massive (you know who you are – 'eoussss'), Mike Ash, Samantha Boyle and Gyles Bailey. Apologies if I have forgotten anyone.

I am grateful to my partners Debbie, Helen and Dan plus the whole team at The Maltings Surgery for being a truly special family of colleagues.

Talking of family, Shai and Michelle – I appreciate your love and support.

Special thanks to my wife Sukie for putting up with an overworked, slightly ungrateful grump for the last eighteen months. You have made this project possible by being selfless and supportive through extraordinary times while keeping your own plates spinning. Love you. May our adventures continue apace.

Reuben and Uma – you both continue to light up our lives. Keep shining.

I must mention and thank my mum, who has had a tough couple of years, for always being there, fussing over us continuously with unconditional love.

Dad would have loved this book and I miss the conversations and debates that we will now never be able to have. I would not have become a medic if it wasn't for mum and dad making it look so easy.

I am a supporter of Leafyard, an app that can help you create changes in your life.
To find out more visit Leafyard.com/healthfix.